The Health Benefits of Vitamins and Minerals

By

Louis N. Chude

Copyright © 2023 by Louis N. Chude - All Rights Reserved.

No part of this eBook may be transmitted or reproduced in any form, including print, electronic, photocopying, scanning, mechanical, or recording, without prior written permission from the author. This e-book has been written for informational purposes only. Every effort has been made to make this eBook as complete and accurate as possible. However, there may be mistakes in typography or content. This e-book provides current information up to the publishing date. As such, it does not include information beyond that date to which the author has subsequently been enlightened.

Table of Contents

Introduction 1
What Are Vitamins? 2
List of 13 Vitamins 5
What Are Fat-Soluble Vitamins? 6
What Are Water-Soluble Vitamins? 8
    Difference between Water-Soluble and Fat-Soluble 10
Importance of Vitamin A (Retinol) 12
    What is Vitamin A? 12
    What are the Benefits of Vitamin A? 13
        Vitamin A Helps to Battle the Free Radicals 13
        Vitamin A Gives Your Face a Younger Appearance 13
        Vitamin A Protects Your Eyes 14
        Vitamin A Helps to Reduce Hyperpigmentation In The Skin 15
        Vitamin A Helps to Reduce the Risk Of Some Particular Cancers 15
        Vitamin A Helps to Reduce the Risk of Acne 16
        Vitamin A Supports the Health of the Bone 18
Importance of Vitamin B1 (Thiamin) 22
    What is Vitamin B1? 22
    What Natural Sources Can You Get Vitamin B1 From? 23
    What are the Benefits of Vitamin B1? 24
        Vitamin B1 Helps to Deal with Sepsis 24
        Vitamin B1 Helps to Boost the Production of Energy 25
        Vitamin B1 Helps to Battle Depression 25

- Vitamin B1 Is Good for Diabetic Patients 25
- Vitamin B1 Helps to Reduce the Risk of Heart Disease .. 26
- Vitamin B1 Helps in Improving Your Memory 27
- Vitamin B1 Helps in The Process of Digestion................ 27

Importance of Vitamin B2 (Riboflavin) 29
- What is Vitamin B2? 29
- What Natural Sources Can You Get Vitamin B2 From? 31
  - Beef Liver 31
  - Breakfast Cereals 32
  - Dairy Products 32
  - Other Sources 32
- What are the Benefits of Vitamin B2? 32
  - Vitamin B2 Helps to Produce Energy 33
  - Vitamin B2 Aids in The Process of Growth and Development 33
  - Vitamin B2 Prevents the Onset of Many Diseases 33
  - Vitamin B2 Is Good for Your Skin 33
  - Vitamin B2 Helps in the regulation of thyroid Activity ... 34
  - Vitamin B2 Helps in The Protection of The Nervous System 34
  - Vitamin B2 Also Helps to Protect Your Vision 34
  - Vitamin B2 Also Helps in The Absorption of Minerals and Vitamins 34

Importance of Vitamin B3 (Niacin) 36
- What is Vitamin B3? 36
- What Natural Sources Can You Get Vitamin B3 From? 37
  - Beef Liver 38

  Fish 38

  Turkey 39

  Pork 39

  Others 40

 What are the Benefits of Vitamin B3? 40

  Vitamin B3 Helps to Keep the Cholesterol Levels in Check 40

  Vitamin B3 May Help in Decreasing the Blood Pressure 40

  Vitamin B3 Helps to Boost the Function Of The Brain ... 41

  Vitamin B3 Helps in Improving the Health of The Skin .. 41

  Vitamin B3 Helps in Regulating the Process of Digestion 42

  Vitamin B3 May Help in The Treatment of Type 1 Diabetes 42

  Vitamin B3 Helps in The Treatment of Pellagra 43

  Vitamin B3 Helps in Reducing the Symptoms of Arthritis 43

  Vitamin B3 May Also Help in Reducing Migraines 43

Importance of Vitamin B5 (Pantothenic Acid) 45

 What is Vitamin B5? 45

 What Natural Sources Can You Get Vitamin B5 From? 46

  Seeds Of Sunflower 46

  Liver 47

  Shiitake Mushrooms 47

  Portobello Mushrooms 47

  Lentils 48

  Fish 48

    Tomatoes (Sun-dried) 48

    Organic Corn 49

    Cauliflower 49

    Eggs 49

    Avocados 49

What are the Benefits of Vitamin B5? 50

    Vitamin B5 Maintains a Healthy Digestive Function 50

    Vitamin B5 Helps in The Conversion of The Food into Energy 50

    Vitamin B5 Helps in Dealing with The Skin Issues 50

    Vitamin B5 Helps in The Synthesis of Coenzyme A 51

    Vitamin B5 Helps in The Lowering the Level Of Cholesterol and Triglycerides 51

    Vitamin B5 Helps to Battle Rheumatoid Arthritis 51

    Ricotta Cheese 53

    Milk 54

    Fish 54

    Liver 55

    Spinach 55

    Carrots 56

What are the Benefits Of Vitamin B6? 56

    Vitamin B6 Helps In Keeping Your Heart Healthy 56

    Vitamin B6 Helps In Reducing The Morning Sickness ... 56

    Vitamin B6 Helps Strengthen The Immune System Of The Body 57

    Vitamin B6 Helps In The Betterment Of The Function Of The Brain 57

Vitamin B6 Helps To Lower The Risk Of Cancer 57

Vitamin B6 Helps In The Betterment Of Mood 57

Vitamin B6 Helps In Dealing With The Effects Of PMS. 58

Importance of Vitamin B7 (Biotin) 59

What is Vitamin B7? 59

What Natural Sources Can You Get Vitamin B7 From? 60

Egg Yolk 60

Liver 61

Avocado 61

Salmon 62

Nuts & Seeds 62

Legumes 62

Sweet Potatoes 62

Yeast 63

What are the Benefits of Vitamin B7? 63

Vitamin B7 Helps in A Stable Pregnancy 63

Vitamin B7 Helps in Managing Diabetes 64

Vitamin B7 Helps in The Improvement of Nails, Hair, And Skin 64

Vitamin B7 Helps to Regulate the Metabolic System 64

Vitamin B7 Promotes the Function of the Brain 65

Importance of Vitamin B9 (Folate) 66

What is Vitamin B9? 66

What Natural Sources Can You Get Vitamin B9 From? 67

Legumes 68

Seeds And Nuts 68

  Broccoli 69

  Asparagus 69

 What are the Benefits of Vitamin B9? 69

  Vitamin B9 Helps In the Treatment of Mental Health Conditions 70

  Vitamin B9 Helps In a Healthy Pregnancy 70

  Vitamin B9 Reduces the Risk of a Heart Attack 70

Importance of Vitamin B12 (Cobalamin) 71

 What is Vitamin B12? 71

 What Natural Sources Can You Get Vitamin B12 From? 72

  Liver and Kidneys 72

  Milk 73

  Shellfish 73

  Fortified Cereals 73

  Fish 74

  Eggs 74

  Yogurt 74

 What are the Benefits of Vitamin B12? 74

  Vitamin B12 Help In Supporting The Skin, Nails, And Hair 75

  Vitamin B12 Helps in Keeping the Heart Healthy 75

  Vitamin B12 Is Linked To the Loss of Neurons in the Brain 76

  Vitamin B12 Is Linked With the Improvement in Depression and Can Also Help Elevate the Mood 77

  Vitamin B12 Can Help In the Prevention of Birth Defects 78

- Vitamin B12 Helps in Supporting the Health of the Bone ... 78
- Importance of Vitamin C (Ascorbic Acid) ... 80
  - What is Vitamin C? ... 80
  - What Natural Sources Can You Get Vitamin C From? ... 81
    - Guavas ... 81
    - Oranges ... 81
    - Plums ... 81
    - Rose Hip ... 81
    - Cherries ... 82
    - Chilli Peppers ... 82
    - Blackcurrants ... 82
  - What are the Benefits of Vitamin C? ... 83
    - Vitamin C Helps In Decreasing The Risk Of Chronic Disease ... 83
    - Vitamin C Manages High Blood Pressure ... 83
    - Vitamin C Prevents Iron Deficiency ... 83
    - Vitamin C Helps in Boosting the Immunity of the Body . 84
    - Vitamin C Helps in Lowering the Risk of Heart Disease . 84
- Importance of Vitamin D (Calciferol) ... 85
  - What is Vitamin D? ... 85
    - Fish ... 86
    - Yolks ... 86
    - Mushrooms ... 87
  - What are the Benefits of Vitamin D? ... 87
    - Vitamin D Helps In Weight Loss ... 87
    - Vitamin D Helps In Battling Depression ... 87

  It May Help In Battling Diseases 88

  It May Help In Supporting the Health of the Immune System 88

Importance of Vitamin E (Tocopherol) 89

  What is Vitamin E? 89

  What Natural Sources Can You Get Vitamin E From? 90

    Beet Greens 90

    Trout 91

    Spinach 91

    Avocados 91

    Almonds 92

    Peanuts 92

    Oils 92

  What are the Benefits of Vitamin E? 93

    Vitamin E Helps in Battling Oxidative Stress 93

    Vitamin E Helps People with NAFLD 93

    Vitamin E Helps To Manage Dysmenorrhea 94

    Vitamin E Help Decrease The Risk Of Heart Disease 94

Importance of Vitamin K (Phylloquinone) 95

  What is Vitamin K? 95

  What Natural Sources Can You Get Vitamin K From? 96

    Kale 96

    Soybeans 96

    Sauerkraut 97

    Asparagus 97

    Lettuce 97

- Broccoli 97
- Brussels sprouts 98
- Turnip greens 98
- Collard greens 98
- Pumpkin 98
- Pickles 99
- Edamame 99
- Blueberries 99
- Pine nuts 99

What are the Benefits of Vitamin K? 99
- Vitamin K Helps in the Healing Of The Wounds 99
- Vitamin K Helps in The Prevention of Osteoporosis 100
- Vitamin K Decreases the Risks of Heart Disease 101
- Vitamin K Helps In Reducing The Blood Pressure 101
- Vitamin K Helps in the Improvement of the Memory of Older Adults 101

How Do Vitamins Work? 103
- The Working of Water-Soluble Vitamins 103
- The Working Of Fat-Soluble Vitamins 104

Importance of Vitamins 105
- Vitamins Are Essential For the Human Body 105
- Why Are These Micronutrients Important? 106
  - Blindness 106
  - Scurvy 106
  - Rickets 107
  - Prevention of Birth Defects 107

Strengthened Bones 107
Maintaining The Health Of Your Teeth 107
What is the need for Vitamin Supplements? 108
Supplements of Vitamin D.. 109
Folic Acid And Pregnancy 109
Vitamin A, C, and D Supplements 109
Are The Supplements of Vitamins A Safe Option? 110
What is Better - Supplements or a Balanced Diet?......... 110
Do Vegetarians Require Supplements? 111
Do Vegans Require Supplements? 111
The Optimum Daily Intake of Vitamins................................ 112
What Are Minerals? 119
Why Are Minerals Important? 121
Essential Minerals That Your Body Needs 122
Calcium 122
Sodium 122
Potassium 123
Chloride.. 123
Magnesium... 123
Phosphorus 124
Iodine 124
Iron... 124
Zinc 125
Copper.. 125
Manganese 125
Sulfur 126

- Selenium 126
- Importance of Calcium 127
  - Functions of Calcium 128
    - Calcium Is Essential For Bone Health 128
    - Calcium Is Essential For the Contraction of Muscles 128
    - Calcium Is Essential For the Clotting Of Blood 129
    - Calcium Maintains Activity of the Heart 129
    - Calcium Also Has Other Benefits 129
  - Signs of Deficiency 130
    - Problems in the Muscles 130
    - They Face Extreme Fatigue 130
    - Problems In the Skin and Nails 130
    - They Suffer From Osteoporosis and Osteopenia 131
    - Severity In PMS 131
    - It Leads to Dental Problems 132
    - It is Linked With Depression 132
  - Signs of Toxicity 132
- Importance of Chromium 133
  - Functions of Chromium 133
    - Chromium Aids in The Metabolism 134
    - Chromium Helps in The Insulin Synthesis 134
    - Chromium Helps in Many Other Functions 134
  - Signs Of Deficiency 135
  - Signs of Toxicity 135
- Importance of Copper 136
  - Functions of Copper 136

- Copper Helps in Maintaining the Cardiovascular Health of the Body 137
- Copper Helps in the signaling of Neurons 137
- Copper Improves the Immune Function of the Body 137
- Copper Reduces the Risk of Osteoporosis 137
- Copper Maintains the Production of Collagen 138
- Copper Deficiency can Lead to Arthritis 138
- Copper May Act as an Antioxidant 138
- Signs of Deficiency 138
- Signs of Toxicity 138

Importance of Fluoride 140
- Functions of Fluoride 140
- Signs of Deficiency 141
- Signs of Toxicity 141

Importance of Iron 142
- Functions of Iron 143
  - Iron Is Essential For The Process Of Cell Division 144
  - Iron Helps in Reducing Fatigue and Tiredness in Humans 144
  - Iron is essential for the cognitive function of the body .. 144
  - Iron helps in performing functions of the immune system 145
  - Iron helps the body in the production of energy 145
  - Iron helps in the transportation of oxygen in the body ... 145
  - Iron helps in the production of red blood cells and hemoglobin 145
- Signs of Deficiency 147

- Pregnancy or Menstruation 147
- Insufficient Intake of Iron 147
- Internal Bleeding 148
- Endometriosis 148
- The Inability of the Body to Absorb Iron 148
- Genetics 148

Importance of Iodine 150
- Functions of Iodine 150
  - It Helps In the Promotion of the Thyroid Health 150
  - It Helps in Reducing the Risk of Certain Goiters 151
  - It Helps In Managing an Overactive Thyroid Gland 151
  - It Helps In the Improvement of the Cognitive Function. 152
  - It Helps In the Development of the Nervous System during Pregnancy 152
  - It Helps In Improving the Birth Weight 153
- Signs of Deficiency 153
- Signs of Toxicity 154

Importance of Magnesium 155
- Functions of Magnesium 155
  - It Helps In the Creation of Energy 155
  - It Helps In the Maintenance of Genes 155
  - It Helps In the Formation of Proteins 155
  - It Helps In Regulating the Nervous System 155
  - It May Help In Battling Depression 155
- Signs of Deficiency 156
- Signs of Toxicity 156

- Importance of Manganese 157
  - Functions of Manganese 157
    - It Helps Produce Enzymes 157
    - It Boosts the Important Systems of The Body 157
    - It Helps In Dealing with Arthritis 157
    - It May Help People With Diabetes 158
    - It Helps In the Metabolism 158
    - It Has Antioxidant Properties 158
  - Signs of Deficiency 158
  - Signs of Toxicity 158
- Importance of Molybdenum 160
  - Functions of Molybdenum 160
  - Signs of Deficiency 161
  - Signs of Toxicity 161
- Importance of Phosphorus 162
  - Functions of Phosphorus 162
    - It Helps In Strengthen the Teeth 162
    - It Helps In the Production of Energy 162
    - It Helps In the Formation of Genetic Material 163
  - Signs of Deficiency 163
  - Signs of Toxicity 163
- Importance of Selenium 164
  - Functions of Selenium 164
    - It Behaves As an Antioxidant 164
    - It Protects Against the Heart Disease 164
    - It May Reduce the Chances of Some Cancers 165

  It Helps In Preventing the Decline of Mental Abilities .. 165
 Signs of Deficiency 165
 Signs of Toxicity 165
Importance of Potassium.. 166
 Functions of Potassium 167
  It Helps In the Regulation of Fluid Balance 167
  It Is Important For the Nervous System 167
  It Helps In the Regulation of Heart and Muscle Contractions.. 167
 Signs of Deficiency 168
 Signs of Toxicity 168
Importance of Zinc... 169
 Functions of Zinc 169
  It Accelerates the Healing Of the Wounds 169
  It May Help In Battling a Couple of Diseases................. 169
  It Helps In Boosting the Immune System 169
 Signs of Deficiency 170
 Signs of Toxicity 170
Bibliography 171

Introduction

Vitamins and Minerals are two important compounds required to keep our body healthy. They help it function in a better manner. Both vitamins and minerals are organic in nature and aid in a wide range of metabolic processes.[1]

We intake vitamins and minerals through the food that we eat on a regular basis. For that purpose, we should focus on eating a balanced and varied diet to reap the benefits of minerals and vitamins from our food.[2] As minerals and vitamins are micronutrients, they tend to make up a really minor portion of our diet. When we are talking about vitamins and minerals, a tiny intake can last you for a long time, so it is not much of a problem.

As you move forth, you will learn in-depth about the vitamins, their thirteen different types, and their functions.

You can also understand the role of vitamin supplements and the correct diet for getting your vitamins.

An elaborate discussion about minerals and the different types of minerals will enable you to understand them much better than before.

---

[1] *APUS: An Introduction to Nutrition (Byerley)*. (2017, June 14). Medicine LibreTexts.
https://med.libretexts.org/Courses/American_Public_University/APUS%3A_An_Introduction_to_Nutrition_(Byerley)

[2] Health benefits of eating well. (2020). NHS Health Scotland.

What Are Vitamins?

In general, vitamins are essential components your body requires to function in a certain way. They are organic in nature and can be found in small quantities in our food.[3] That is why a balanced diet is very important; it helps you to get your vitamins. This, in turn, will keep your body functioning in a stable and healthy manner.

The human body produces low amounts of certain vitamins, but the rest should be fulfilled through the food we eat.

When we talk about vitamins, we need them in an adequate amount - if we intake a lesser amount of vitamins, it will result in a deficiency, and if you consume too many vitamins, it will result in toxicity - and both conditions can lead to different kinds of health issues.

While being organic, the vitamins tend to contain carbon.

The vitamin requirement of each and every organism varies quite significantly.

When humans require Vitamin C, we must get it from our diets.

Contrary to this, whenever the dogs require excess Vitamin C, they produce it naturally with the help of their glandular system. When we take a healthy dog as an example, it will produce around 18mg of Vitamin C for each pound of weight it possesses.[4] Suppose the dog weighs 50 pounds; this would mean it will produce around 900 mg of vitamin C in one day. This will enable

---

[3] Brazier Y. (2020). Vitamins: What are they, and what do they do? Medicalnewstoday.com

[4] Rabe J. (2017). How Dogs Produce Vitamin C. https://animals.mom.com/how-dogs-produce-vitamin-c-12332800.html

the dog's system to get an ongoing concentration of ascorbic acid throughout the day.

Some vitamins cannot be found in sufficient amounts in the food. Instead, you can find them in other natural sources. For example, when our body is exposed to sunlight, this allows the body to synthesize vitamin D. Hence, sunlight is considered the best source to get your dose of Vitamin D.

All vitamins work to play various different roles, and the body requires a different amount of all the vitamins in order to stay healthy.

Vitamins offer many important benefits to the body. If your bones are strong, it is due to Vitamin D that is present in your body.[5]

Vitamin A is the best when it comes to improving the vision of your body.[6]

Vitamin C efficiently aids in healing the wounds in your body.[7]

---

[5] *Vitamin D for Good Bone Health - OrthoInfo - AAOS*. (n.d.). Www.orthoinfo.org. https://orthoinfo.aaos.org/en/staying-healthy/vitamin-d-for-good-bone-health/

[6] *4 essential vitamins for eye health*. (2022, May 13). Www.medicalnewstoday.com. https://www.medicalnewstoday.com/articles/326758#:~:text=Vitamin%20A%20is%20essential%20for

[7] Chambial, S., Dwivedi, S., Shukla, K. K., John, P. J., & Sharma, P. (2013). Vitamin C in Disease Prevention and Cure: An Overview. *Indian Journal of Clinical Biochemistry*, *28*(4), 314–328. https://doi.org/10.1007/s12291-013-0375-3

Vitamin B12 is adept at transforming the food that you intake into energy.[8]

Different vitamins offer your body the functional support it requires.

---

[8]Vitamin B12 (Cobalamin) Information | Mount Sinai - New York. (n.d.). Mount Sinai Health System. https://www.mountsinai.org/health-library/supplement/vitamin-b12-cobalamin

List of 13 Vitamins

1. Vitamin A - It is also known as Retinol
2. Vitamin B1 - It is also known as Thiamin
3. Vitamin B2 - It is also known as Riboflavin
4. Vitamin B3 - It is also known as Niacin
5. Vitamin B5 - It is also known as Pantothenic Acid
6. Vitamin B6 - It is also known as Pyridoxine
7. Vitamin B7 - It is also known as Biotin
8. Vitamin B9 - It is also known as Folate or Folic Acid
9. Vitamin B12 - It is also known as Cobalamin
10. Vitamin C - It is also known as Ascorbic Acid
11. Vitamin D - It is also known as Calciferol
12. Vitamin E - It is also known as Tocopherol
13. Vitamin K - It is also known as Phylloquinone

These thirteen vitamins are further broken down into two categories:

1. Fat-soluble vitamins
2. Water-soluble vitamins

What Are Fat-Soluble Vitamins?

You can find the vitamins falling under two types of categories based on their solubility; one is water-soluble vitamins. The second category is the one that we are going to discuss - they are fat-soluble vitamins.

Fat-soluble vitamins are found in abundance in foods that are high in fats. When you consume fats from food, it enables the fat-soluble vitamins to absorb into your body.[9]

The vitamins that are absorbed in your body in such a manner pave their way to the fat tissues of the body and liver and are accumulated there. The storage of your fat-soluble vitamins can last for an extended period of time. When they are reserved in the fat tissues of the body, they can easily be stored for around six months. If your body requires fat-soluble vitamins, it utilizes them from the stored stocks in the fat tissues of the body.

The fat-soluble vitamins are not able to be absorbed in water. [10]Amongst all the vitamins, the four fat-soluble vitamins are:

1. Vitamin A
2. Vitamin D
3. Vitamin E
4. Vitamin K

While they are very beneficial when consumed in adequate proportions, the toxicity of fat-soluble vitamins leads to higher

---

[9] Fletcher, J. (2020, January 17). Fat-soluble vitamins: Types, function, and sources.www.medicalnewstoday.com.
https://www.medicalnewstoday.com/articles/320310
[10]The Fat-Soluble Vitamins: A, D, E and K. (2017, February 16). Health line. https://www.healthline.com/nutrition/fat-soluble-vitamins#:~:text=Vitamins%20can%20be%20classified%20based

risk as compared to water-soluble vitamins. [11] For that purpose, consuming a well-balanced diet is essential. If you are taking supplements for Vitamin A, D, E, or Vitamin K, make sure to consult your doctor beforehand to reduce the chance of toxicity.

Some diseases like Cystic Fibrosis, Chronic Pancreatitis, and IBD (Inflammatory Bowel Disease) can cause reduced absorption when it comes to fat; this results in a decreased absorption of Vitamin A, Vitamin D, Vitamin E, and Vitamin K as well. [12] This can cause a deficiency of vitamins. Hence, it is important that you get in touch with a medical professional regarding it and look out for any potential problems that can occur in your health.

---

[11] Fat-Soluble Vitamins: A, D, E, and K - 9.315 - Extension. (2018). Extension. https://extension.colostate.edu/topic-areas/nutrition-food-safety-health/fat-soluble-vitamins-a-d-e-and-k-9-315/

[12] *Fat-Soluble Vitamins: A, D, E, and K - 9.315 - Extension.* (2018). Extension. https://extension.colostate.edu/topic-areas/nutrition-food-safety-health/fat-soluble-vitamins-a-d-e-and-k-9-315/

What Are Water-Soluble Vitamins?

As the name suggests, these are vitamins that can dissolve in water. These help the body function properly. When the water-soluble vitamins enter the body, they are shifted to the tissues of the body through the bloodstream. However, they are not stored in the body. After the body has utilized the required supply, the water-soluble vitamins are excreted through the urine. [13]

As the water-soluble vitamins are excreted out on a regular basis, it is mandatory to replenish them frequently. You can find water-soluble vitamins in many plants and animals. A well-balanced diet allows the intake of water-soluble vitamins.

Vitamin C and the range of B vitamins fall in the category of water-soluble vitamins. [14]

The nine water-soluble vitamins are vitamin C and the collection of other B vitamins, including:

1. Vitamin C
2. Vitamin B1
3. Vitamin B2
4. Vitamin B3
5. Vitamin B5
6. Vitamin B6

---

[13] Vitamin - The water-soluble vitamins | Britannica. (2019). In *Encyclopædia Britannica*.
https://www.britannica.com/science/vitamin/The-water-soluble-vitamins
[14] Lykstad, J., & Sharma, S. (2022). Biochemistry, Water Soluble Vitamins. PubMed; StatPearls Publishing.
https://www.ncbi.nlm.nih.gov/books/NBK538510/#:~:text=The%20water%2Dsoluble%20vitamins%20include

7. Vitamin B7

8. Vitamin B9

9. Vitamin B12

Even though the above-mentioned vitamins are classified as water-soluble, the degree of solubility in water varies. The degree of solubility in water of these water-soluble vitamins influences the pathway of absorption, determines their excretory pathways, and provides a clear distinction between water-soluble vitamins and fat-soluble vitamins.[15]

These vitamins contain some elements like carbon, oxygen, hydrogen, etc. Some vitamins even contain cobalt, sulfur, or nitrogen.

When the water-soluble vitamins are present in their so-called free states, they are inactive.[16] For them to be activated, they are supposed to be with their respective coenzyme forms.

Thiamin, Pyridoxine, and Riboflavin are activated by adding phosphate groups. As the phosphate group is added, they undergo a shift in the structure that leads to the activation of Biotin.

A complex compound is formed amidst the part of other molecules and the free vitamin. This activates pantothenic acid, niacin, folic acid, and cobalamin.

---

[15] Lykstad, J., & Sharma, S. (2020). Biochemistry, Water Soluble Vitamins. PubMed; StatPearls Publishing.
https://www.ncbi.nlm.nih.gov/books/NBK538510/

[16] Vitamin - The water-soluble vitamins | Britannica. (2019). In *Encyclopædia Britannica*.
https://www.britannica.com/science/vitamin/The-water-soluble-vitamins

After the formation of the active coenzyme, it should merge with the appropriate protein component (termed an apoenzyme) that allows enzyme-catalyzed reactions to occur. [17]

Difference between Water-Soluble and Fat-Soluble

To make a comparison between the water-soluble vitamins and the fat-soluble vitamins, we have provided a chart below. It will help you understand the basic points in which water-soluble vitamins differ from fat-soluble vitamins.[18]

Water-Soluble Vitamins	Fat-Soluble Vitamins
As per the name, water-soluble can only be dissolved in water.	As per the name, Fat-Soluble Vitamins can be dissolved in fat.
Examples of Water-soluble vitamins are Vitamin B (and all its types) and Vitamin C.	Examples of Fat-Soluble Vitamins are Vitamin A, Vitamin D, Vitamin E, and Vitamin K.
Water-Soluble Vitamins are hydrophilic in nature.	Fat-Soluble Vitamins are hydrophobic in nature.
The excessive Water-Soluble Vitamins are passed through the kidney and excreted through urine.	Excessive Fat-Soluble Vitamins are reserved in the fatty tissues of the body.

---

[17] Blanco, A., & Blanco, G. (2016). *Enzymes - an overview | ScienceDirect Topics*.Sciencedirect.com.
https://www.sciencedirect.com/topics/neuroscience/enzymes
[18] Alma, L. (2018). *What Is the Difference Between Fat-Soluble and Water-Soluble Vitamins?* Verywell Health. https://www.verywellhealth.com/fat-vs-water-soluble-998218

Water-Soluble Vitamins are able to travel in the bloodstream freely.	Fat-Soluble Vitamins stand in need of a carrier protein that helps them in transportation around the blood.
The abundance of Water-Soluble Vitamins is not very toxic as compared to Fat-Soluble Vitamins.	The abundance of Fat-Soluble Vitamins can be more toxic as compared to Water-Soluble Vitamins.
The symptoms of deficiency when it comes to Water-Soluble Vitamins are quickly visible.	The symptoms of deficiency when it comes to Fat-Soluble Vitamins take time to manifest.

Importance of Vitamin A (Retinol)

What is Vitamin A?

Vitamin A is also called Retinol. It is an important nutrient that aids in supporting skin, reproductive health, eye, and immune functions.

You can get Vitamin A from various animal products. Sources of Vitamin A are meat, dairy, and poultry.

They are even found in plant products, which means that you can find them in many vegetables and fruits.

It is the job of your liver to convert Vitamin A to retinol. After it is converted, the retinol is stored in the liver, and the lymphatic system transports it to the cells throughout the body.

The human skin is responsive to retinoids and can easily absorb them when applied topically.

What Natural Sources Can You Get Vitamin A From?

You can find Vitamin A in many foods like dairy products or spinach. Food rich in beta-carotene also works as an excellent source of Vitamin A as your body converts beta-carotene into vitamin A. [19]

Many leafy vegetables are rich in beta-carotene. [20]For example, you can find beta-carotene in broccoli, spinach, and kale. It can also be found in orange and yellow vegetables, for instance,

---

[19] Olsen, N. (2018, February 7). *Benefits of Beta Carotene and How to Get It*. Healthline; Healthline Media.
https://www.healthline.com/health/beta-carotene-benefits

[20] *Beta-carotene Information | Mount Sinai - New York*. (n.d.). Mount Sinai Health System. https://www.mountsinai.org/health-library/supplement/beta-carotene#:~:text=Dietary%20Sources

carrots, pumpkins, sweet potatoes, summer squash, and winter squash.

Other sources to get your Vitamin A are red tomatoes, red bell peppers, beef liver, fish oils, mangoes, cantaloupes, milk, fortified foods, and eggs.

What are the Benefits of Vitamin A?

Vitamin A Helps to Battle the Free Radicals
Vitamin A also consists of antioxidant properties.[21] Vitamin A's antioxidant properties help combat the effect of free radicals. Free radicals are those particular molecules produced when the food is broken down in the body or your body is exposed to some environmental aggressors, like tobacco, smoke, or radiation. These free radicals can result in potentially dangerous outcomes like heart disease or cancer.

Vitamin A efficiently helps to battle against these free radicals.[22]

Vitamin A Gives Your Face a Younger Appearance
Using Vitamin, A topically can stimulate collagen production, reducing the early onset of wrinkles, fine lines, and skin sagging.[23] This helps your skin to have a younger appearance.

The collagen boost also helps improve the skin's elasticity and keeps the skin firm and youthful.[24] It also helps to promote angiogenesis.

---

[21] Mayo Clinic Staff. (2020, November 13). *Vitamin A*. Mayo Clinic. https://www.mayoclinic.org/drugs-supplements-vitamin-a/art-20365945
[22] Better Health Channel. (2012). Antioxidants. Vic.gov.au. https://www.betterhealth.vic.gov.au/health/healthyliving/antioxidants
[23] *What Can Vitamin A Do for Your Skin?* (2022, March 25). Healthline. https://www.healthline.com/health/beauty-skincare/vitamin-a-for-skin
[24] *8 ways to stimulate collagen production in skin*. (2017, April 26). Www.medicalnewstoday.com. https://www.medicalnewstoday.com/articles/317151

Vitamin A Protects Your Eyes

If you want to preserve your eyesight, Vitamin A is necessary for that. The body requires this vitamin to convert the light that reaches the eye and transforms it into an electrical signal transmitted to the brain.

If you have a deficiency of Vitamin A, you can also suffer from nyctalopia or night blindness. The deficiency of Vitamin A causes night blindness because Vitamin A is a vital component of a pigment named rhodopsin.[25]

Rhodopsin can be found in the eye, specifically in the retina, and it is considered particularly sensitive to light.[26]

People going through this condition can see perfectly during the day, but their vision at night becomes flawed due to the strain on their eyes.

Other than night blindness, you can also slow down the upcoming eye-light deterioration by eating food enriched with beta carotene.

The leading reason for blindness is AMD or Age-related macular degeneration.[27] While the exact reason for this is still not known, it is presumed that Age-related macular degeneration results due to the cellular damage that is caused to the retina due to oxidative stress.

---

[25] *The Mechanism for Vitamin A Improvements in Night Vision.* (2015). Ebmconsult.com. https://www.ebmconsult.com/articles/vitamin-a-eye-vision-mechanism

[26] Rogers, K. (2019). Rhodopsin | biochemistry. In *Encyclopædia Britannica.* https://www.britannica.com/science/rhodopsin

[27] Age-Related Macular Degeneration. (n.d.). WebMD. https://www.webmd.com/eye-health/maculardegeneration/age-related-macular-degeneration overview#:~:text=Age%2Drelated%20macular%20degeneration%20(AMD

Including Beta-Carotene in the diet can help improve your eyesight and save you from many eye-related diseases.[28]

Vitamin A Helps to Reduce Hyperpigmentation In The Skin
If your diet contains a sufficient amount of carotenoids, for instance, beta carotene, it will reduce cell damage and skin aging.[29] Carotenoids are known for their ability to protect the skin from environmental aggressors like the harmful rays of the sun and pollution.[30]

This helps improve the appearance and health of the skin in a positive way.

Vitamin A promotes cellular turnover, which assists in battling hyperpigmentation, dark spots, sun spots, and aging signs, and helps you get an even skin tone. [31]

Vitamin A Helps to Reduce the Risk Of Some Particular Cancers
The abnormal growth of cells causes cancer. The cells undergo rapid growth or abnormal division, leading to cancer.

Vitamin A is an important component in the development and growth of the body's cells; hence, it influences the prevention of cancer.

---

[28] Benefits of Beta Carotene and How to Get It. (2020, July 30). Health line. https://www.healthline.com/health/beta-carotene benefits#:~:text=Diets%20rich%20in%20carotenoids%20like

[29] *Health Benefits of Beta Carotene.* (n.d.). WebMD. https://www.webmd.com/diet/health-benefits-beta-carotene

[30] Baswan, S. M., Klosner, A. E., Weir, C., Salter-Venzon, D., Gellenbeck, K. W., Leverett, J., & Krutmann, J. (2021). Role of ingestible carotenoids in skin protection: A review of clinical evidence. Photodermatology, Photoimmunology & Photomedicine, 37(6), 490–504. https://doi.org/10.1111/phpp.12690

[31] *Vitamin A: The Skincare Benefits of Retinoids | NUME-Lab.* (n.d.). NUME-Lab Switzerland. Retrieved August 16, 2022, from https://www.nume-lab.com/vitamin-a-for-skin/

According to observational studies, it has been seen that consuming an increased amount of Vitamin A (especially in the form of beta-carotene) has been seen to reduce the onset of some particular cancers. These cancers include cervical cancer, lung cancer, bladder cancer, and Hodgkin's lymphoma.[32]

This is mainly observed in the increased consumption of vitamin A, particularly from plants rather than animal sources.

Even the Vitamin A supplements did not show the results that reached the plant-based ones.

While the exact mechanism is still not fully worked out, according to current evidence, it is safe to say that vitamin A is considered to be healthy for cell division and can lead to a reduced risk for some particular kinds of cancers.

Vitamin A Helps to Reduce the Risk of Acne
People who have suffered from acne are trying countless remedies, medications, etc., to get rid of it. Acne is basically a skin disorder that is considered to be chronic and also inflammatory.

People going through this condition tend to develop spots (that can sometimes be painful), whiteheads, and blackheads primarily located on their chest, face, and back. The clogged-up sebaceous glands cause these spots. The sebaceous glands become clogged with grease, dirt, and dead cells.

These glands increase the production of sebum which is a waxy component that keeps the skin waterproof and also lubricated.

---

[32] West, H. (2018, August 23). *6 Health Benefits of Vitamin A, Backed by Science.* Healthline; Healthline Media.
https://www.healthline.com/nutrition/vitamin-a-benefits

Acne is not really hazardous to health, but it can have a bad effect on a person's self-esteem and can be a reason for anxiety and depression.

While the exact relation between Vitamin A and acne has not been concluded, it is quite prominent that a decrease in the levels of Vitamin A can trigger the onset of acne.[33]

The deficiency of Vitamin A results in an overproduction of keratin in the follicles of hair.[34] This causes an increased risk of acne as the dead skin cells accumulate in the hair follicles and lead to blockages.

Some medications for acne are even based on vitamin A to battle acne in a consistent manner. The name of one oral retinoid is Isotretinoin, which is known to be highly effective in dealing with severe acne. You need to take it under medical supervision as it can have negative effects if not prescribed accurately.

Vitamin A Helps to Treat Psoriasis

The topical and oral medications of Vitamin A are known to treat psoriasis. The raised patches of psoriasis can be calmed by the topical retinoid.

You can also be prescribed some oral medications by your healthcare adviser to deal with severe psoriasis.

---

[33] El-akawi, Z., Abdel-Latif, N., & Abdul-Razzak, K. (2006). Does the plasma level of vitamins A and E affect acne condition? *Clinical and Experimental Dermatology, 31*(3), 430–434.
https://doi.org/10.1111/j.1365-2230.2006.02106.x

[34] Petre, A. (2019, November 4). *8 Common Signs of Vitamin Deficiency, Plus How to Fix Them*. Healthline.
https://www.healthline.com/nutrition/vitamin-deficiency

Some drugs infused with Vitamin A are used to deal with cutaneous T-cell lymphoma - skin cancer that causes excessive rashes, major itching, and dryness.[35]

So, in general, Vitamin A serves well to deal with your skin diseases as well.

Vitamin A Supports the Health of the Bone
As we have learned from the beginning, the vital components for maintaining healthy and strong bones are calcium, Vitamin D, and protein. [36]

While it is not a vital component for the health of bone, however, the consumption of Vitamin A in adequate amounts is mandatory for the development and growth of strong bones.

It has been observed that a deficiency of Vitamin A can result in poor condition of bone health.

People with insufficient levels of Vitamin A in their blood levels are at an increased risk of fractures of the bones compared to people with healthy levels of Vitamin A.

With that being said, the decreased amount of vitamin A is not the only concern when we are talking about the health of the bone. According to some studies, an increased amount of vitamin A has also resulted in a risk of fractures.

---

[35] *What Can Vitamin A Do for Your Skin?* (2022, March 25). Healthline. https://www.healthline.com/health/beauty-skincare/vitamin-a-for-skin
[36] *Calcium and bones: MedlinePlus Medical Encyclopedia.* (2016). Medlineplus.gov. https://medlineplus.gov/ency/article/002062.html

An Overview of Vitamin B Complex

The B complex vitamins are an essential group of nutrients that are deemed essential by the body. They help in playing important roles in the functioning of the body. You can find them in many food products and consume them in many forms. Many foods are fortified with B Complex Vitamins. Also, you may find them in supplement form as well.

Due to so many foods containing B-complex Vitamins, it is comparatively easier to get them into your diet. Due to many factors, you may require more B Vitamins than before. This includes age, diet, pregnancy, genetics, medical conditions, and the use of alcohol. Due to these, your doctor or healthcare professional may prescribe B-complex supplements to you.

B-complex vitamins are water-soluble in nature. This [37] means that they can be dissolved in the blood. They are not stored in the blood; instead, they are excreted out of the body through urination. Hence, you should be careful about maintaining an adequate diet that has a consumption of B-complex vitamins on a regular basis.

The B vitamins play a direct role in the maintenance of good health. They help in enabling you to have a healthy body; due to this, they also directly affect the metabolism of cells, the function of the brain, and the level of energy you possess.

---

[37] Water-Soluble Vitamins: B-Complex and Vitamin C - 9.312. (n.d.). Extension.
Retrieved August 16, 2022, from https://extension.colostate.edu/topic-areas/nutrition-food-safety-health/water-soluble-vitamins-b-complex-and-vitamin-c-9-312/#:~:text=B%2Dcomplex%20vitamins%20and%20vitamin

They also help in preventing the body from infectious diseases and help in promoting many other functions as well. They play a supporting role in maintaining cell health, red blood cell growth, levels of energy, the sight of the eye, the function of the brain, and digestive functions. They also help in promoting your appetite. Furthermore, they ensure the proper function of the nerves and hormones. Other than that, Vitamins of the B-complex reduce bad cholesterol levels and help keep cardiovascular health and muscle tone in check.

Why Have The B-Complex Vitamins Grouped Together?

All the Vitamins in the B-complex consist of loose similarities in their properties. Along with this, similarities can also be seen in the distribution of the natural sources, and even their functions are seen to be overlapping extensively. Due to this, they are placed in a broader group of B-complex vitamins.

Other than that, while vitamins A, D, E, and K are known to be fat-soluble, all the vitamins of the B-complex, along with Vitamin C, are water-soluble.

There are B vitamins that have been identified as coenzymes as they take action along with the enzymes and work to accelerate the conversion of the chemical compounds. They also help in participating in the metabolic functions that take place in the body.

The B-complex vitamins include:

Vitamin B1, also known as Thiamine.

Vitamin B2, also known as Riboflavin.

Vitamin B3, also known as Niacin.

Vitamin B5, also known as Pantothenic acid.

Vitamin B6, also known as Pyridoxine.

Vitamin B7, also known as Biotin.

Vitamin B9, also known as Folate.

Vitamin B12, also known as Cobalamin.

All the B-vitamins combine to be known as the B-complex vitamins. [38]

---

[38] *https://www.cancer.gov/publications/dictionaries/cancer-terms/def/vitamin-b-complex*. (2011, February 2). Www.cancer.gov.
https://www.cancer.gov/publications/dictionaries/cancer-terms/def/vitamin-b-complex

Importance of Vitamin B1 (Thiamin)

What is Vitamin B1?

Vitamin B1 is also called Thiamin. Thiamin is a vitamin that permits your body to utilize carbohydrates and use them as a source of energy.[39] This is done by thiamin as it is required by the body to make ATP (adenosine triphosphate). Hence, ATP helps in the transportation of energy.

Thiamin holds immense importance in many functions, for example, the function of the heart, nerves, muscles, and the metabolism of glucose. Thiamin is required by your tissues to help them work in an orderly manner.

Thiamin was named Vitamin B1 because it was the very first Vitamin B that was discovered by scientists.[40]

Vitamin B1 is a water-soluble vitamin and can be easily dissolved in water. These water-soluble vitamins are transported through the bloodstream. A small portion of Vitamin B1 is stored in the liver. Excessive leftovers are excreted by the body in the form of urine.

Due to this reason, you need to get a diet rich in thiamin on a daily basis. You can get Vitamin B1 from natural food, fortified food, and multivitamins.

---

[39] *Vitamin B1 (Thiamine) Information | Mount Sinai - New York.* (n.d.). Mount Sinai Health System.
https://www.mountsinai.org/health-library/supplement/vitamin-b1-thiamine

[40] *Vitamin B1 (Thiamine) Information | Mount Sinai - New York.* (n.d.). Mount Sinai Health System.
https://www.mountsinai.org/health-library/supplement/vitamin-b1-thiamine

What Natural Sources Can You Get Vitamin B1 From?

The body does not store Vitamin B1 (except for a very small amount stored in your liver). Due to this reason, you need to intake Vitamin B1 on a daily basis so that you can keep the functions of the body running at a smooth pace. Make sure that you intake a proper level of Vitamin B1 in your daily routine so that the excretion of the excess levels does not mess up the requirement by your body to carry out its activities.

You get thiamin from many natural sources. Other than that, thiamin is also added to a couple of food items, so you can also obtain it from them.

You can obtain a good Thiamin concentration from the cereals' outermost layers. Vitamin B1 can also be found in pork, yeast, whole grains, pulses, beef, fish, lentils, and nuts.[41]

Some fruits are enriched with Vitamin B1, too; these include oranges, grapes, jackfruit, pineapple, raisins, avocado, grapefruit, figs, currants, and cantaloupe. Other fruits containing Vitamin B1 are blueberry, watermelon, apricot, plums, cherries, honeydew, nectarine, raspberries, mango, and kiwi.

Some vegetables are rich in Vitamin B1 too, and they include green beans, summer squash, carrots, onions, tomatoes, cauliflower, green peas, kale, broccoli, asparagus, and potatoes.

Blackstrap molasses are also a good source of Vitamin B1.

There are some breakfast products like cereals that may also contain vitamin B1. Processing of the food results in destroying

---

[41] Harvard T.H. Chan. (2019, July 8). *Thiamin – Vitamin B1*. The Nutrition Source. https://www.hsph.harvard.edu/nutritionsource/vitamin-b1/

the thiamin. [42]Vitamin B1 is found in both kinds of rice, that is, white rice and brown rice. However, white rice that is not fortified with Vitamin B1 will contain only one-tenth of the thiamin levels that are found in brown rice.

A single piece of whole wheat bread consists of 0.1 mg of Vitamin B1. It adds up to seven percent of the daily thiamine requirement.

You will not find any thiamin in apples, chicken, or cheese. If you are a noodle lover, you would be happy to know that you can also gain your thiamine doses from noodles. Apart from that, you can also find Vitamin B1 in yogurt and sunflower seeds.

What are the Benefits of Vitamin B1?

Vitamin B1 Helps to Deal with Sepsis
When you get an infection, it has the ability to trigger a chain reaction that can cause problems in your body. Sepsis can turn out to be quite fatal if your body does not have a sufficient amount of Vitamin B1. Vitamin B1 and Vitamin C join hands to battle sepsis and save your body from the severe response that can occur due to the infection.

[43]Sepsis can also result in renal failure. Hence due to low Vitamin B1 levels, you can even risk kidney failure.

With adequate levels of Vitamin B1 in your body, you can fight sepsis and keep your body in a condition to battle any added infection.

---

[42] Thiaminase - an overview | ScienceDirect Topics. (n.d.). Www.sciencedirect.com. Retrieved October 7, 2022, from https://www.sciencedirect.com/topics/biochemistry-genetics-and-molecular-biology/thiaminase

[43] Contributors, W. E. (2021, June 23). *Health Benefits of Vitamin B1*. WebMD. https://www.webmd.com/vitamins-and-supplements/health-benefits-of-vitamin-b-1

Vitamin B1 Helps to Boost the Production of Energy

When we intake nutrients in our body, vitamin B1 works to break down and free the energy that is acquired from the diet. Whatever levels of lipids, carbohydrates, and lipids we consume are converted into energy with the help of Vitamin B1; due to this, Vitamin B1 is important when it comes to energy.

The merge between the levels of sugar and Vitamin B1 in your body consequently forms energy. Thiamin aids in accelerating this procedure and also lends its support to the enzymes.

Vitamin B1 Helps to Battle Depression

There is a strong connection between Vitamin B1 and depression. Lower levels of Vitamin B1 are connected to having an inactive mood. The intake of Vitamin B1 supplements is a good source that can help you battle depression.

With thiamin, a change was observed in people having a major depressive disorder. The signs of depression started to ameliorate. [44]This is the reason why Vitamin B1 is considered a potential cure for people suffering from depression.

Hence, you need to ensure that you are getting proper levels of thiamin on a daily basis. [45]This will help you keep yourself safe from mental problems like depression, stress, and anxiety.

Vitamin B1 Is Good for Diabetic Patients

For people who are diabetic, getting an adequate quantity of vitamin B1 is very important. According to studies, if you consume vitamin B1 consistently for a time span of six weeks, this will result in an improvement in insulin levels as well as blood

---

[44]*Depression, aggression, and Vitamin B1 thiamine supplements as a new treatment.* (2019, November 18). Eat2BeNice. https://newbrainnutrition.com/depression-aggression-and-vitamin-b1-thiamine-supplements-as-a-new-treatment/

[45] National Institutes of Health. (2017). *Office of Dietary Supplements - Thiamin.* Nih.gov. https://ods.od.nih.gov/factsheets/Thiamin-HealthProfessional/

sugar levels.[46] Not only this, but Thiamin also aids in a decrease in complications in heart and blood pressure.

Thiamin is an essential component for the metabolism of glucose. The low level of thiamin in diabetic patients can cause a severity in the initial stages of diabetes.

Apart from that, Vitamin B1 also helps to reduce the problems of kidneys in people suffering from Type 2 diabetes.

In a study on diabetic patients, it was observed that the people who had type 1 or type 2 diabetes also showed a lower range of thiamin levels than the people who were not suffering from diabetes.[47] People with diabetes can often experience nerve pains, thiamin also aids in curing those nerve pains, and this can even result in no need for a painkiller.

Vitamin B1 Helps to Reduce the Risk of Heart Disease

Along with its many functions, Vitamin B1 also helps to reduce the risk of a disease of the heart. Acetylcholine is produced with the presence of Thiamin. [48]Due to this, your body is able to convey messages between the muscles and nerves. If there is any gap in this communication, it will cause problems in the working of your heart. Hence insufficient levels of Vitamin B1 are linked with problems in cardiac function. [49]

---

[46] Alaei Shahmiri, F., Soares, M. J., Zhao, Y., & Sherriff, J. (2013). High-dose thiamine supplementation improves glucose tolerance in hyperglycemic individuals: a randomized, double-blind cross-over trial. *European journal of nutrition, 52*(7), 1821-1824.

[47] Anwar, A., Ahmed Azmi, M., Siddiqui, J. A., Panhwar, G., Shaikh, F., & Ariff, M. (2020). Thiamine Level in Type I and Type II Diabetes Mellitus Patients: A Comparative Study Focusing on Hematological and Biochemical Evaluations. *Cureus*. https://doi.org/10.7759/cureus.8027

[48] Mann, P. J. G., & Quastel, J. H. (1940). Vitamin B1 and Acetylcholine Formation in Isolated Brain. *Nature, 145*(3683), 856–857. https://doi.org/10.1038/145856a0

[49] Ao, M., Yamamoto, K., Ohta, J., Abe, Y., Niki, N., Inoue, S., Tanaka, S., Kuwabara, A., Miyawaki, T., & Tanaka, K. (2019). Possible involvement of thiamine insufficiency in heart failure in the institutionalized elderly. *Journal of Clinical Biochemistry and Nutrition, 64*(3), 239–242. https://doi.org/10.3164/jcbn.18-85

Make sure that you have a proper supply of Vitamin B1 on a daily basis so that it does not cause you any risk related to the heart.

Vitamin B1 Helps in Improving Your Memory

Low levels of vitamin B1 can result in a deficit in memory. With proper thiamine in your system, you will experience an improvement in your memory as well as concentration. Thiamin is known to have a positive influence on your brain function as well as attitude.[50]

Vitamin B1 Help in Lowering the Risk of Cataracts

According to studies, it is suggested that sufficient levels of Vitamin B1 can also aid in reducing the probability of developing cataracts. It was observed that the people who had consumed a large amount of protein in combination with vitamins in their food had a lower chance of developing cataracts. Getting your proper dose of vitamins can help to protect your eyes and also the lens of the eye.

Vitamin B1 Helps in The Process of Digestion

To save yourself from the problems occurring in the process of digestion, you need to maintain proper levels of vitamin B1 in your diet. Hydrochloric acid is needed by the body to help in the maintenance of proper digestive function, and the production of hydrochloric acid is regulated by Vitamin B1. [51]

If there are low levels of vitamin B1, it will not be able to regulate hydrochloric acid thoroughly, which would result in indigestion.

---

[50] Contributors, W. E. (2021, June 23). *Health Benefits of Vitamin B1*. WebMD. https://www.webmd.com/vitamins-and-supplements/health-benefits-of-vitamin-b-1

[51] https://www.pharmaca.com/projectwellness/the-scoop-on-vitamins-vitamin-b1-thiamine/

Hence, if you want to get effective digestion without any problems, you need to get an adequate amount of Vitamin B1 in your diet.

Importance of Vitamin B2 (Riboflavin)

What is Vitamin B2?

Vitamin B2 is also known as Riboflavin. It is in the list of the 8 B vitamins that are termed important for the health of humans. You can get Vitamin B2 from many things like plants, grains, and even dairy products. Riboflavin is quite essential to breaking down the components of food, aiding in the absorption of nutrients, and also helping in the maintenance of the tissues. [52]

Like all the other Vitamin B vitamins, Vitamin B2 is also water-soluble. This means that it can dissolve in water too. It is transported through the bloodstream, and when they are utilized, they are excreted out of the body through the urine.

Due to this, only a small amount of Vitamin B2 is stored by the body, and the rest is all excreted out of the body. Hence you require a daily dose of Vitamin B2 to keep up the levels of Riboflavin maintained.

If you do not intake Vitamin B2 on a daily basis, this will result in a downfall of the supply. Riboflavin can be ingested in three forms, it can be obtained in its natural forms, it can be added to food, or it can also be taken in the form of supplements.

The bacteria that are present in the gut are also able to produce a minute amount of Vitamin B2, but that amount is insufficient to meet dietary needs.

Riboflavin in the body is absorbed in the small intestine.

The B Vitamins are altogether termed B-complex vitamins. All the B-complex vitamins aid the body in the production of energy by aiding in the conversion of carbohydrates (food) into

---

[52] *Riboflavin – Vitamin B2*. (2020, July 24). The Nutrition Source. https://www.hsph.harvard.edu/nutritionsource/riboflavin-vitamin-b2/

glucose (fuel). They also aid in metabolizing proteins and fats. You need to keep the supply of B-complex vitamins proper in order to have a properly functioning liver, hair, eyes, and skin.[53] Other than that, the B-complex vitamins also assist the nervous system in functioning in a proper way.

Vitamin B2 is an essential element of the coenzymes that work towards cell growth, production of energy, fat breakdown, steroid breakdown, and the breakdown of medications.

While your body excretes the excess Vitamin B2 levels through urine, sometimes the body can contain excessive riboflavin through their diets or supplements. This can be hinted at by the color of urine; when there is an excess of vitamin B2 in the body, the color of the urine will turn bright yellow.[54]

Vitamin B2 is also important because it also aids in changing vitamin B6 (pyridoxine) and folate into forms that are usable by the body. [55]Other than that, it also aids in the production and growth of the RBCs (red blood cells).

Most people can get sufficient amounts of riboflavin through the intake of a proper and well-balanced diet. As people get older, they might be at risk of deficiency of riboflavin.[56] Other than that, alcoholics are also at risk of deficiency in Vitamin B2 due to their poor dietary conditions.

---

[53] Sarwar, M. F., Sarwar, M. H., & Sarwar, M. (2021). Deficiency of Vitamin B-Complex and Its Relation with Body Disorders. In *www.intechopen.com*. IntechOpen. https://www.intechopen.com/chapters/78374

[54] *Riboflavin - Health Encyclopedia - University of Rochester Medical Center*. (n.d.). Www.urmc.rochester.edu.
https://www.urmc.rochester.edu/encyclopedia/content.aspx?contenttypeid=19&contentid=vitaminb-2

[55] https://www.verywellfit.com/b-complex-vitamins-89411

[56] Amber, A.-M. (2011, June 8). *Riboflavin Diet | How to Age Less | Look Great | Live Longer | Health and Lifestyle*. Slow Aging | Healthy Living, Healthy Aging. https://slowaging.org/vitamin-b2-and-aging/

If someone has a deficiency of Vitamin B2, they will experience the following symptoms:

- They would feel fatigued and tired.
- They would experience slow growth.
- The tongue would be swollen, and the color would be a little toward the magenta shade.
- The eyes would experience fatigue.
- They would also suffer from digestive problems.
- There are cracks and sores that are visible around the corners of the mouth.
- They would experience issues with light sensitivity.
- They would experience a sore throat.
- They would experience swelling in the throat.

What Natural Sources Can You Get Vitamin B2 From?

You can find Vitamin B2 in many natural sources. Other than that, you can also obtain it from fortified food or from supplements. Some food that is rich in Vitamin B2 are:

Beef Liver
The beef liver is enriched with riboflavin and is known as one of the richest natural sources of Vitamin B2. [57]You can intake 2.9 mg of Vitamin B2 just from eating three ounces of

---

[57] *Is beef liver good or bad for you?* (n.d.). Heartstone Farm. Retrieved October 9, 2022, from https://www.heartstonefarm.me/blogs/about-grass-fed-beef/is-beef-liver-good-or-bad-for-you

cooked liver. The figure sums up to twice the requirement of your body.

Breakfast Cereals

When it comes to breakfast cereals, many of them are fortified with B-complex vitamins, including Vitamin B2. [58]If you are consuming a proper serving of breakfast cereal that is fortified with Vitamin B2, this will allow you to get your daily recommended value of Vitamin B2 from it.

Dairy Products

You can get your daily intake of Vitamin B2 through milk and yogurt as well.[59]

Other Sources

Other than this, clams also have vitamin B2. If you love a clambake, that is good for your vitamin B2 levels. People who are vegetarians can also get their Vitamin B2 levels sorted from the mushrooms.

Almonds have been known as a great source of protein and fiber, but they also have Vitamin B2! You can get Vitamin B2 from eggs as well.

Fortified tofu, Salmon, Lean Pork Chops, Avocados, and Spinach also contain some level of Vitamin B2 in them.

If you are a cheese lover, you would be happy to know that you can get your intake of Vitamin B2 from it as well.

Turkey, chicken, beef, and fish all contain Vitamin B2. [60]

What are the Benefits of Vitamin B2?

---

[58] McCulloch, M. (2018, October 11). *15 Healthy Foods High in B Vitamins*. Healthline; Healthline Media. https://www.healthline.com/nutrition/vitamin-b-foods

[59] *Riboflavin – Vitamin B2*. (2020, July 24). The Nutrition Source. https://www.hsph.harvard.edu/nutritionsource/riboflavin-vitamin-b2/

[60] https://www.rxlist.com/vitamin_b2/definition.htm

Vitamin B2 has several benefits for health, some of which are stated below.

Vitamin B2 Helps to Produce Energy
Vitamin B2 helps in the breakdown of carbohydrates, proteins, and fats that help in producing energy. Hence, riboflavin plays an important role in giving a little boost to energy levels.

Vitamin B2 Aids in The Process of Growth and Development
Riboflavin is very important as it helps in the process of development and growth. It makes sure that there is proper growth of the tissues of the body, like skin, eyes, mucous membranes, connective tissues, the immune system, and the nervous system.

It also deals with the development of reproductive organs. Apart from that, it also makes sure that your nails, hair, and skin are healthy.

Vitamin B2 Prevents the Onset of Many Diseases
Vitamin B2 is very important in stopping the onset of many health-related problems. It can help to deal with many problems like headaches, acne, dermatitis, cataracts, arthritis, migraine, eczema, and rheumatoid arthritis.

Hence, low levels of Vitamin B2 can have an effect on many things.

Vitamin B2 Is Good for Your Skin
Adequate levels of Vitamin B2 are very important on a daily basis to keep our skin in good condition. Riboflavin is a vitamin that helps in giving your skin an improved appearance. [61]This is done by giving a brighter and dewy look to your face. It also helps your skin to create a perfect balance between the natural oils. These vitamins are really beneficial for skin, whether it is acne-prone skin or dry skin. Vitamin B2 works wonders on all.

---

[61] *The Journal.* (n.d.). AVEENO®. Retrieved October 9, 2022, from https://www.aveeno.com/journal/all-ways-vitamin-b-skin-sooo-gaood

Vitamin B2 Helps in the regulation of thyroid Activity

Vitamin B2 is important to carry out the activity done in the thyroid. [62]If there is a lack of Riboflavin, it will result in suppressing the function of the thyroid, which in turn will result in a problem. If the function of the thyroid is not working perfectly, it would consequently cause the adrenal glands not to secrete the hormones.

Vitamin B2 Helps in The Protection of The Nervous System

Vitamin B2 also keeps your nervous system protected. It does this by generating a feeling of relief when a person undergoes extreme levels of anxiety. It is also seen that when Vitamin B2 is merged with Vitamin B6, it effectively deals with the symptoms caused by carpal tunnel syndrome (CTS) and treats them.

Vitamin B2 Also Helps to Protect Your Vision

When it comes to vision, Vitamin B2 plays an important part in it. It makes sure that the corneas are healthy. Also, they also make sure that you have a perfect vision. Other than that, Vitamin B2 is essential to protect you from getting cataracts. Hence, you need to make sure that you get a good diet on a daily basis that contains the required levels of Vitamin B2.

Vitamin B2 Also Helps in The Absorption of Minerals and Vitamins

Vitamin B2 is important in dealing with the absorption of minerals. [63] It helps in the absorption of a variety of minerals like folic acid and iron and assists the absorption of other vitamins like Vitamin B1, Vitamin B2, and Vitamin B6.

Regular intake of Vitamin B2 is important for the proper absorption of minerals and vitamins.

---

[62] *Thyroid Nutrition*. (n.d.). Sunwarrior. Retrieved October 9, 2022, from https://sunwarrior.com/blogs/health-hub/thyroid-nutrition

[63] Brazier, Y. (2017, March 7). *Vitamin B2: Role, sources, and deficiency.* Www.medicalnewstoday.com. https://www.medicalnewstoday.com/articles/219561

Importance of Vitamin B3 (Niacin)

What is Vitamin B3?

Vitamin B3 is a vitamin that is also known as Niacin. It is an important part of the B-complex and is a vitamin that is water-soluble in nature, which means that it can be dissolved in water.

You can get it from three sources; the first one is through naturally occurring sources - food, you can get it from fortified food, and you can also get it through your supplements. When it comes to Niacin, you can find three different forms of Vitamin B3 in your supplements and food, the first one being nicotinic acid, the other one is called nicotinamide, and the third form is nicotinamide riboside. [64]

The body has the ability to make a conversion of tryptophan (that is, an amino acid) to nicotinamide. These three types of Vitamin B3 are transformed into the body to integrate Nicotinamide Adenine Dinucleotide (i.e., NAD), and it is extremely difficult to get NAD without any of the B3 vitamins or an essential amino acid tryptophan.

The extra amount of Niacin in the body that is not required by the body is not stored; it is excreted out of the body through urine. Niacin is essential for our body as it acts as a coenzyme - and that makes it an essential component for more than 400 enzymes. This denotes the fact that more than 400 enzymes are reliant on Niacin to perform their due functions. Other than that, Niacin also helps in the conversion of different carbohydrates into energy, repairs and creates DNA, creates fats and cholesterol, and also helps in exerting the effects of antioxidants.

---

[64]Harvard School of Public Health. (2020, July 6). *Niacin – Vitamin B3*. The Nutrition Source.
https://www.hsph.harvard.edu/nutritionsource/niacin-vitamin-b3/

What Natural Sources Can You Get Vitamin B3 From?

The easiest way to intake this essential Vitamin is through the foods that you ingest. Others take an alternate route and take the help of supplements to keep their supply of this beneficial Vitamin sufficient. While some also have to take the help of prescription niacin that would aid them in different medical conditions, the most common one being high levels of cholesterol.

The two most common forms of Niacin are niacinamide (also known as nicotinamide) and nicotinic acid. Both these types are available in your niacin supplements as well as food.

Since Niacin is excreted by the urine and no storage is done, it is mandatory that you get a regular supply of this Vitamin. You have to ingest a diet that is rich in vitamin B3 or take supplements to help your body get sufficient levels of Vitamin B3.

Here are a few foods that have Vitamin B3 in them.

Here are 16 foods high in Niacin:

Chicken Breast

While the entire chicken is good for your intake of Vitamin B3, chicken breast takes the lead in providing the maximum nutrient as compared to the entire chicken[65].

If we consider three ounces of cooked chicken breast that is also skinless and without bones, you will be getting a total of 11.4 mg of Vitamin B3 through it.

This would sum up to 81% of the total Recommended Dietary Allowance for females and 71% of it for males.

---

[65] *Top Foods High in Niacin*. (n.d.). WebMD. https://www.webmd.com/diet/foods-high-in-niacin-b3#1

If we consider three ounces of the chicken thigh that does not have bones and is skinless, they will be providing half the amount comparatively.

Other than the niacin levels, chicken breast is also an excellent source of protein.

Beef Liver

Consuming cooked liver is excellent for giving a little boost to your niacin levels. [66]The liver is enriched with Vitamin B3.

When a man consumes three ounces of beef liver in the cooked form, they will be able to ingest a total of 14.7 mg of Vitamin B3. This means that they will be consuming around 91% of the required Vitamin B3 just by eating 3 ounces of cooked liver. For women, the three ounces would surpass the 100% RDA levels.

Hence, the cooked liver is termed an excellent source of Vitamin B3.

Note: *Other than Vitamin B3, the liver is stacked with other nutrients as well. You can get iron, protein, Vitamin A, choline, and also other B-Complex vitamins from it.*

Fish

Tuna and Salmon are both considered good sources when it comes to Niacin. [67]People who like eating fish can benefit from it.

If you use a 165 g of tuna can as an example, it is going to give you 21.9 mg of Niacin. This will be more than 100 percent of the Recommended Dietary Allowance for women and men.

Other than Niacin, tuna is also enriched with protein, pyridoxine, selenium, cobalamin, etc.

---

[66] Julson, E. (2018). *16 Foods That Are High in Niacin (Vitamin B3)*. Healthline. https://www.healthline.com/nutrition/foods-high-in-niacin

[67] Julson, E. (2018). *16 Foods That Are High in Niacin (Vitamin B3)*. Healthline. https://www.healthline.com/nutrition/foods-high-in-niacin

Other than Tuna, Salmon is also considered a good option to get your supply of Niacin. If you cook three ounces of Salmon filet, it will provide you with 61% of the Recommended Dietary Allowance for women and 53% for men.

Apart from Niacin, Salmon is termed an excellent source of omega-3 fatty acids.

Note: *Wild Salmon is a better option than farmed Salmon.* [68]

Turkey
Turkey has a bit of a twist to it; rather than having a larger niacin level, it helps to provide tryptophan. This tryptophan is utilized by the body and converted into Niacin.[69] When we consider 3 ounces of turkey breast that is cooked, it will be providing around 6.3 mg of Niacin, which can be added by one more mg due to the presence of tryptophan.

This will suffice for 46% of the Recommended Dietary for men and 52% of it for women.

Pork
Other than turkey, chicken, and beef, pork also adds to the list of food that gives you Niacin. Pork chops and pork tenderloin are considered good sources of Vitamin B3.

Eating three ounces of pork chops will give you 6.3 mg of Vitamin B3. According to the RDA, this will make up 45% of the required levels for women and 39% of the required levels for men.

Pork is also considered a good source of Vitamin B1.

---

[68] Julson, E. (2018). *16 Foods That Are High in Niacin (Vitamin B3)*. Healthline. https://www.healthline.com/nutrition/foods-high-in-niacin

[69] *Tryptophan: MedlinePlus Medical Encyclopedia*. (2013). Medlineplus.gov. https://medlineplus.gov/ency/article/002332.htm

Others

There are many other sources of Vitamin B3 as well. It includes green peas, mushrooms, whole wheat, peanuts, avocados, brown rice, potatoes, etc.

It is found in many foods that are plant-based as well as animal-based. Some more sources include eggs, nuts, dairy, legumes, bread, seed, and fortified cereals.

What are the Benefits of Vitamin B3?

Vitamin B3 Helps to Keep the Cholesterol Levels in Check
When you are prescribed medication to decrease your cholesterol levels, sometimes they also suggest Niacin with it. [70]This aids in normalizing the lipid levels in the blood. It is done by Niacin, as it is thought to increase the level of healthy cholesterol (HDL cholesterol - high-density lipoprotein) by a margin of 15% to 35%.

At the same time, it works to decrease the levels of bad cholesterol (LDL cholesterol - Low-density lipoprotein) by a margin of 5% to 25%.

This also helps battle the risk of heart attack along with low-density lipoprotein cholesterol; this also decreases triglycerides.

Vitamin B3 May Help in Decreasing the Blood Pressure
Vitamin B3 performs an active role in releasing prostaglandin. [71]These are chemicals that help to dilate the blood vessels, that in turn increase the flow of blood and hence reduce the blood

---

[70]*Niacin to boost your HDL, "good," cholesterol.* (2018). Mayo Clinic. https://www.mayoclinic.org/diseases-conditions/high-blood-cholesterol/in-depth/niacin/art-20046208

[71] Kwong, A. M., Tippin, B. L., Materi, A. M., Buslon, V. S., French, S. W., & Lin, H. J. (2011). High dietary niacin may increase prostaglandin formation but does not increase tumor formation in ApcMin/+ mice. *Nutrition and Cancer*, *63*(6), 950–959. https://doi.org/10.1080/01635581.2011.590266

pressure. Due to this ability, this Vitamin is thought to be essential in battling the problems linked with high blood pressure.

In a case study, it was observed that if you increased the quantity of Niacin by 1 mg on a regular basis, it would result in a decrease in high blood pressure risk by 2%.

This needs more scientific data to back it up and prove it for now.

Vitamin B3 Helps to Boost the Function Of The Brain
Vitamin B3 is essential to carry out some functions of the brain. For instance, your brain requires Vitamin B3 to activate the function of the coenzymes NADP and NAD - both of them are dependent on Niacin to function in a proper manner. Proper functioning of the coenzymes NAD and NADP would result in the production of energy.

Other than this, there are some psychiatric symptoms that are closely linked with the deficiency of Vitamin B3.

Niacin can help in the treatment of some specific types of Schizophrenia - this is done by reversing the damage that has been done to the brain cells as a result of the deficiency of Niacin.

According to some studies, Vitamin B3 can also aid in keeping the brain healthy. [72]

Vitamin B3 Helps in Improving the Health of The Skin
Vitamin B3 plays an important role in keeping your skin healthy. If you use Vitamin B3 orally or in the form of lotions, it will help in the protection of the cells of your skin against harmful UV rays. [73]

---

[72] Contributors, W. E. (2021, June 23). *Health Benefits of Vitamin B1*. WebMD. https://www.webmd.com/vitamins-and-supplements/health-benefits-of-vitamin-b-1

[73] Cherney, K. (2018, August 28). *Everything You Should Know About Niacinamide*. Healthline; Healthline Media.
https://www.healthline.com/health/beauty-skin-care/niacinamide

Vitamin B3 is also used in many skincare products to boost the level of hydration in the skin and make it soft, supple, and plumper. Niacin is known to be a part of many anti-aging cosmetics as it deals with fine lines, wrinkles and skin sagging and helps you in attaining younger and more gorgeous skin.

Other than that, Niacin also helps to battle dark spots and hyperpigmentation and therefore helps you in achieving even-toned skin.

A study suggests that Vitamin B3 helps in preventing your skin from cancer. This is not proven yet, but much research points toward this.

Vitamin B3 Helps in Regulating the Process of Digestion
Niacin is an essential component for the normal working of the digestive system of humans. This affects your skin and appetite in a positive manner - it makes your appetite healthy and gives a glowing radiance to your skin. An important component for the function of the digestive system, this Vitamin helps in the breakdown of carbohydrates, alcohol, and fats. Hence, you can get your digestion problems sorted in an easy manner if they are due to niacin deficiency.

Vitamin B3 May Help in The Treatment of Type 1 Diabetes
In Type 1 diabetes, your body starts to attack and destroy the cells that are creating insulin in your pancreas. Hence, it is termed an autoimmune disease. Children are more prone to this condition. According to research, Vitamin B3 is active in the protection of these cells, and due to this, they help in lowering the risk of type 1 diabetes in children. [74]

---

[74]Cabrera-Rode, E., Molina, G., Arranz, C., Vera, M., González, P., Suárez, R., Prieto, M., Padrón, S., León, R., Tillan, J., García, I., Tiberti, C., Rodríguez, O. M., Gutiérrez, A., Fernández, T., Govea, A., Hernández, J., Chiong, D., Domínguez, E., & Di Mario, U. (2006). Effect of standard nicotinamide in the prevention of type 1 diabetes in first degree relatives of persons with type 1 diabetes. *Autoimmunity*, *39*(4), 333–340.
https://doi.org/10.1080/08916930600738383

Vitamin B3 Helps in The Treatment of Pellagra
Pellagra is termed a disease that is due to the deficiency of Niacin in the human body. [75]Due to this, they may experience symptoms like depression, confusion, headaches, apathy, anxiety, mood changes, irritability, disorientation, or even delusions.

Other than these, some people may even experience soreness on their tongues, gum, or lips. Some face a severe decrease in appetite, or they feel nauseated and end up vomiting. Some people face trouble drinking and eating the bare minimum.

As a treatment, the patients have been prescribed an adequate intake of Niacin through supplements as well as their diet. They are suggested to increase the food that contains Niacin in it so that they can get rid of all the symptoms.

Vitamin B3 Helps in Reducing the Symptoms of Arthritis
Several results have been observed where Vitamin B3 has been showing signs of reducing the symptoms of arthritis. It helps in increasing the mobility of the joints. This allows the freedom to move your hand as per your requirements.

It also works to decrease the inflammatory symptoms that are linked with arthritis due to its anti-inflammatory properties. This has been proving to have a soothing effect on people who are suffering from arthritis.

However, if you take anything in an excessive amount, it can have negative effects on your body. The same is the case with Vitamin B3. An excessive intake of Vitamin B3 can result in problems in health.

Vitamin B3 May Also Help in Reducing Migraines
As per some studies, Vitamin B3 is enriched with therapeutic properties that help in providing relief against migraines and

---

[75] Megan Dix RN-BSN. (2017, December 22). *Pellagra*. Healthline; Healthline Media. https://www.healthline.com/health/pellagra

headaches. [76]It is reasoned to dilate the intracranial vessel, which helps in preventing headaches and migraine.

---

[76] Prousky, J., & Seely, D. (2005). The treatment of migraines and tension-type headaches with intravenous and oral niacin (nicotinic acid): systematic review of the literature. *Nutrition Journal, 4*(1). https://doi.org/10.1186/1475-2891-4-3

Importance of Vitamin B5 (Pantothenic Acid)

What is Vitamin B5?

Vitamin B5 is also named Pantothenic Acid or Pantothenate. Vitamin B5 is a vitamin that comes in the category of water-soluble. [77]This means that it can be dissolved in water.

Pantothenic is a word that is derived from the Greek language. "Pantou" means "everywhere."

This vitamin is an essential vitamin and is deemed important for the proper functioning of humans. Due to this, blood cells are made in the body. Other than that, it has many other functions, too; for instance, it aids in converting your ingested food (fats, carbohydrates, and proteins) to energy.

It has many other functions too.

It helps in keeping your eyes, hair, and skin healthier. Other than that, it is essential for the proper functioning of the liver and nervous system, along with keeping the digestive tract healthy. Vitamin B5 also efficiently helps in the making of red blood cells. In the adrenal glands, pantothenic acid works to make stress-related and sex hormones.

---

[77]*Vitamin B5: Everything you need to know.* (n.d.). Www.medicalnewstoday.com. https://www.medicalnewstoday.com/articles/219601

What Natural Sources Can You Get Vitamin B5 From?

Vitamin B5 is a part of B-complex vitamins that are water-soluble in nature. With water-soluble properties, they can easily dissolve in the blood. The excess amount of vitamin B5 is not stored in the body; they are excreted by the body through the process of urination. [78]Pantothenic acid is very important for a wide variety of functions of the body. Hence, it is necessary to obtain adequate levels of pantothenic on a regular basis so that the functions of the body are not disrupted.

You can obtain Pantothenic Acid from different sources. It is present in many natural foods, it is also added to some foods, or you can also get supplements of pantothenic acid to fix your vitamin B5 levels. There is a bacteria located in your gut that is responsible for the production of pantothenic acid, but the quantity is very low, and hence, it is not sufficient to meet the requirements of the diet of humans. [79]

Some of the natural sources of pantothenic acid are mentioned below.

Seeds Of Sunflower
Sunflower seeds are a widely popular snack that is tasty, easy as well as stacked with important nutrients like protein, Vitamin B5 and Vitamin E. [80]If you ingest foods that have Vitamin E, it is

---

[78]*Vitamin B5: Everything you need to know.* (n.d.). Www.medicalnewstoday.com.
https://www.medicalnewstoday.com/articles/219601
[79] Boston, 677 H. A., & Ma 02115 +1495-1000. (2020, August 11). *Pantothenic Acid – Vitamin B5.* The Nutrition Source.
https://www.hsph.harvard.edu/nutritionsource/pantothenic-acid-vitamin-b5/
[80] Valente, D. L., M.S., & RD. (n.d.). *4 Amazing Health Benefits of Sunflower Seeds.* EatingWell. Retrieved October 9, 2022, from https://www.eatingwell.com/article/2059940/sunflower-seeds-nutrition/

researched that it helps in decreasing the risk of coronary heart disease by a huge margin.

If you consume three ounces of these sunflower seeds, you will be able to get 6 mg of Vitamin B5 through it.

Liver
You can get Vitamin B5 from the liver of chicken, beef, and even duck. When you talk about Vitamin B levels, the liver is the best source for them.

If you intake three ounces of cooked chicken liver, you will be getting around 8.3 mg of Vitamin B5. Chicken liver has an impressive presence of vitamin B5.

Due to the presence of Vitamin B5 and B12, the cooked chicken liver, when ingested, serves as a really good source for the prevention of anemia.

When you go out to buy the liver, you need to make sure that the chicken is free-range, fed on grass, and raised on pasture.

Shiitake Mushrooms
These shiitake mushrooms are beneficial due to their wide range of nutrients. With the delicious taste, you can also get your Vitamin B5 levels sorted through them. [81]They also have the presence of Vitamin B5 in them. If you consume four dried shiitake mushrooms, you will be able to get around 66% of the recommended dietary allowance for the day.

Hence, this is a good option to add if you want to add to your levels of Vitamin B5.

Portobello Mushrooms
If you ingest one whole cup of portobello mushrooms in sliced forms, this will make up 19 percent of the Recommended Dietary

---

[81] Elaine. (n.d.). *Vitamin B5 (Pantothenic Acid): 8 Shiitake Mushrooms (140g) A Day*. Retrieved October 9, 2022, from http://www.familyfecs.com/2016/04/vitamin-b5-pantothenic-acid-8-shiitake.html

Allowance. The portobello mushrooms are enriched with potassium which helps to regulate the balance of electrolytes as well as the levels of hydration. These mushrooms are rich in all B Vitamins, including Vitamin B5. Hence, the intake of portobello mushrooms can help elevate the level of Vitamin B5 in the body.

Lentils

Lentils are a very good source of health as they have a rich amount of B vitamins along with other nutrients like manganese and folate.

If you use 1 cup of lentils in your diet, you will get around 1.3 mg of Vitamin B5. Lentils are also a good source of protein that is plant-based. [82]For vegetarians, it is best if they incorporate lentils into their diet to get their respective protein intake.

Fish

Eating fish is very beneficial for your health. Eating Salmon that is wild-caught is good as it contains many essential nutrients along with a high quantity of pantothenic acid. [83]

If you consume three ounces of Salmon, it will round off to 1.6 mg of Vitamin B5. Pantothenic acid has anti-inflammatory properties and is also rich in omega-3 fatty acids. Eating Salmon is really beneficial for your health due to its properties.

Tomatoes (Sun-dried)

The ripe tomatoes go through the process of drying out, which gets rid of the water content. One cup of sun-dried tomatoes contains 1.1 mg of Vitamin B5. It also helps decrease issues like cataracts due to the presence of lutein and zeaxanthin.

---

[82] Khazaei, H., Subedi, M., Nickerson, M., Martínez-Villaluenga, C., Frias, J., & Vandenberg, A. (2019). Seed Protein of Lentils: Current Status, Progress, and Food Applications. *Foods, 8*(9), 391. https://doi.org/10.3390/foods8090391

[83] *Top 10 Foods Highest in Vitamin B5 (Pantothenic Acid)*. (n.d.). Myfooddata. https://www.myfooddata.com/articles/foods-high-in-pantothenic-acid-vitamin-B5.php

Organic Corn

If you ingest 1 cup of organic corn that is non-GMO, it means that you will be getting 1.2 mg of Vitamin B5. Eating corn is a healthy option as it is enriched with essentials like complex carbohydrates, fiber, and antioxidants. [84]With the influx of GMO corn, we need to make sure that the corn that we intake is non-GMO.

Cauliflower

If you eat 1 cup of cauliflower, it will give you around 0.7 mg of pantothenic acid. This vegetable is cruciferous and is linked to being able to prevent the onset of cancer.[85]

This vegetable helps in the process of detoxification and digestion due to the glucosinolates - it contains sulfur, which also supports the absorption of nutrients and aids in the removal of wastes.

Eggs

If you consume three ounces of eggs, they will give you 0.9 mg of Vitamin B5. Along with vitamin B5, eggs are also rich in proteins. When you eat eggs that are free range, this will help you in gaining all the essential nutrients from it. It also has omega-3s and beta-cholesterol, though it has fewer amounts of cholesterol.

Avocados

If you eat one fruit of avocado, it will give you around 2 mg of pantothenic acid. It has good levels of Vitamin B5 and is stacked with Vitamin B6. Along with these, it also has monounsaturated fats.

---

[84] Atli Arnarson, PhD. (2019, May 16). *Corn 101: Nutrition Facts and Health Benefits*. Healthline; Healthline Media. https://www.healthline

[85] *Cruciferous Vegetables and Cancer Prevention*. (2010). National Cancer Institute; Cancer.gov.
https://www.cancer.gov/about-cancer/causes-prevention/risk/diet/cruciferous-vegetables-fact-sheet

Avocados have shown positive results on the heart as well as lipid profiles. [86]

What are the Benefits of Vitamin B5?

Pantothenic acid has many important functions in the body.

Vitamin B5 Maintains a Healthy Digestive Function
Pantothenic acid is an essential vitamin. It works to make the digestive system healthy and allows the body to utilize other vitamins like Vitamin B2. [87]The absorption of Vitamin B2 allows the body to manage the levels of stress. So, indirectly, Vitamin B5 helps in dealing with stress too.

Vitamin B5 Helps in The Conversion of The Food into Energy
One of the most important functions of pantothenic acid is to help the human body to convert the ingested food into a source of energy for our body. This vitamin aids the carbs, proteins, and fats to convert into energy that is to be used by the body.

Vitamin B5 Helps in Dealing with The Skin Issues
According to a few studies, pantothenic acid, when used on the skin, behaves as a moisturizer and makes the skin soft and supple. [88]Other than that, it also hastens up the process of healing the wounds. When taken in the form of supplements, pantothenic acid helped in reducing acne and significantly got rid of the blemishes too.

---

[86] Pacheco, L. S., Li, Y., Rimm, E. B., Manson, J. E., Sun, Q., Rexrode, K., Hu, F. B., & Guasch-Ferré, M. (2022). Avocado Consumption and Risk of Cardiovascular Disease in US Adults. *Journal of the American Heart Association*. https://doi.org/10.1161/jaha.121.024014

[87] Morris, R. (2014, December 2). *What Does Vitamin B5 Do?* Healthline; Healthline Media. https://www.healthline.com/health/vitamin-watch-what-does-b5-do

[88] Instagram, A. (n.d.). *Dermatologists Want You to Use Panthenol with Your Hyaluronic Acid Products*. Byrdie. https://www.byrdie.com/panthenol-for-skin-the-complete-guide-4770218

Vitamin B5 Helps in The Synthesis of Coenzyme A
Pantothenic acid plays a leading role in the synthesis of Coenzyme A. Coenzyme A helps to convert food into cholesterol and fatty acids. Coenzyme A is also responsible for the production of sphingosine, a fat-like molecule that aids in delivering chemical messages across the cells of the body.[89]

The liver also requires Coenzyme A for the safe metabolism of toxins and drugs.

If Coenzyme A is not synthesized due to the absence of Vitamin B5, it can lead to a lot of problems in the body.

Vitamin B5 Helps in The Lowering the Level Of Cholesterol and Triglycerides
According to some case studies, it has been shown that pantothenic acid is responsible for lowering the levels of fats and triglycerides that are found in the blood. This method can only be done under the observation of medical professionals.

Vitamin B5 Helps to Battle Rheumatoid Arthritis
According to some research, it showcases that vitamin B5 is lower in people who are suffering from rheumatoid arthritis.[90] Studies are going on to confirm this theory.

---

[89] *Sphingolipid - an overview | ScienceDirect Topics.* (n.d.). Www.sciencedirect.com. Retrieved October 9, 2022, from https://www.sciencedirect.com/topics/agricultural-and-biological-sciences/sphingolipid

[90] *About Vitamin B5: A Guide to Usage and Dosage.* (2016, May 5). Dr. Lam Coaching - World Renowned Authority on Adrenal Fatigue Recovery. https://www.drlamcoaching.com/blog/about-vitamin-b5/

Importance of Vitamin B6 (Pyridoxine)

What is Vitamin B6?

Vitamin B6 is also known as pyridoxine. It is a part of the B-complex vitamins and has water-soluble properties. This means that it is able to absorb easily in the water. It is present in many foods and can also be taken in the form of supplements like capsules, liquid, or tablets. The active coenzyme is called PLP - Pyridoxal 5' Phosphate and is found to be the most significant in the B6 levels of the blood.

PLP is very important for the body as it helps around a hundred enzymes to perform their functions in an effective manner. This includes protein breakdown, carbohydrate breakdown, and fat breakdown. It also helps in the maintenance of adequate levels of homocysteine. The maintenance of homocysteine is very important as high levels can cause problems for the heart. PLP also offers support to the health of the brain and the function of the immune system.

The deficiency of Vitamin B6 often causes kidney disease or problems in the absorption of nutrients. [91] Some causes of Vitamin B6 deficiency revolve around epilepsy medicines and dependence on alcohol, and some autoimmune disorders.

The lack of Vitamin B6 can be dangerous as it would cause a deficiency of red blood cells, which would result in anemia, depression, confusion, and a weak immune system.

---

[91] *Vitamin B6 Deficiency - Disorders of Nutrition.* (n.d.). MSD Manual Consumer Version.
https://www.msdmanuals.com/home/disorders-of-nutrition/vitamins/vitamin-b6-deficiency

What Natural Sources Can You Get Vitamin B6 From?

Pyridoxine, or Vitamin B6, is a component of the B-complex vitamins. This vitamin is very important as it helps in many functions of the body. It helps decrease stress levels along with the maintenance of proper health. [92]It is water-soluble and is dissolved in water. The body does not store Vitamin B6 in the body - like the rest of the B-complex vitamins. The excess Vitamin B6 is excreted out of the body through the urine.

It is necessary to keep a regular intake of Vitamin B6 so that you do not face a deficiency of it as you move forth.

Pyridoxine is a vitamin that is seen to be lacking in diets usually. Hence, you can either try to take them through your supplements. The natural way is considered the best, though, and you can get the levels of Vitamin B6 up with the help of some natural food that is enriched with Vitamin B6.

Ricotta Cheese

If you are a cheese lover, you would be happy to know that you can get your vitamin B6 through ricotta cheese. [93]This water-soluble vitamin is found in the cheese - more specifically in the whey protein content. As the whey levels in the cheese increase, so does the B6 levels. Whey is also sacked with other nutrients like Vitamin B1 (thiamin), folate, Vitamin B3 (niacin), and Vitamin B2 (Riboflavin). Ricotta cheese has the highest amount of whey. Hence it is the highest source of Vitamin B6 when it comes to cheese.

---

[92] National Institutes of Health. (2017). *Office of Dietary Supplements - Vitamin B6*. Nih.gov. https://ods.od.nih.gov/factsheets/vitaminB6-healthprofessional/

[93] *Best 15 Vitamin B-6 Foods: Benefits and Recipes*. (2017, May 26). Healthline. https://www.healthline.com/health/vitamin-b6-foods

Milk

A deficiency of Vitamin B6 can result in a lot of serious problems in health. If you do not have adequate levels of Vitamin B6 in your body, you can face problems in the central nervous system. Milk is a good source of Vitamin B6 and helps to keep its levels of it sorted. [94]

If you consume 1 cup of goat or cow's milk, it will give you 5% of the recommended daily allowance of Vitamin B6. You can also choose low-fat or skim milk; those are also nutritious.

Milk is also beneficial as it helps to provide high levels of calcium and vitamin B12. You can also pair up the milk with fortified cereal and down the milk in this way.

Fish

Salmon is a fish that is healthy for the heart and consists of the largest value of Pyridoxine found in foods. Hence, Salmon is termed an excellent source of Vitamin B6. Pyridoxine is incredibly important for the proper functioning of the adrenal glands. [95]If the adrenal glands are not working perfectly, it will result in a negative impact on cortisol, aldosterone, and adrenalin levels in the body. Adrenal glands are responsible for the regulation of blood pressure and help in keeping blood sugar in check.

Intake of Salmon is very good for health as it is low-fat, nutritious, and rich in proteins. You can find Salmon easily in most restaurants. Wild Salmon are better as they have a higher level of pyridoxine. You can make it as per your convenience and

---

[94] *Best 15 Vitamin B-6 Foods: Benefits and Recipes*. (2017, May 26). Healthline. https://www.healthline.com/health/vitamin-b6-foods

[95](2022). Oup.com. https://academic.oup.com/ajcn/article-abstract/7/4/426/4730002?redirectedFrom=fulltext

taste, experiment with a variety of spices, and broil, sauté, bake or stir-fry them as per your taste.

If you do not like to consume Salmon, you can opt for tuna. Be sure that you are getting the correct ones - albacore and yellowfin tuna.

Tuna has high levels of Vitamin B6 in it, especially in the previously mentioned ones. If you are consuming a tuna steak, you will be able to get the highest concentrations of pyridoxine. Canned tuna also has a good amount of Vitamin B6.

Tuna and Salmon are both rich in omega-3 fatty acids, and this is very beneficial for the development of your brain health.

Liver

The cooked chicken liver is brimming with nutrition. It is stacked with folate, proteins, Vitamin A (retinol), Vitamin B12 (cobalamin), as well as Vitamin B6 (pyridoxine). It is a very good source of nutrition and should be consumed to keep your body functioning in an orderly manner. Due to pyridoxine, your proteins undergo breaking down and are used in the body. The best part about chicken liver is that it is not that expensive. Hence it can be used by everyone. Use it with seasonings that suit your taste buds, and add some pepper and salt to enhance the taste; throw in some onions and green peppers and eat them up for a healthy boost.

Note: Overcooking the liver can make the texture rubbery, so avoid it.

Spinach

Vitamin B6 helps in the production of antibodies that can help battle diseases and infections. You can get the level of antibodies boosted with the help of spinach. Spinach is enriched with Vitamin B6, Vitamin A, and also Vitamin C. [96]It also has iron in

---

[96] Gunnars, K. (2015). *Spinach 101: Nutrition Facts and Health Benefits*. Healthline. https://www.healthline.com/nutrition/foods/spinach

it. Hence, the consumption of spinach will prove to be healthy for your body.

Carrots

Carrot also contains Vitamin B6. Along with this, they are also rich in Vitamin A (Retinol) and fiber. You can use them in juice forms or eat them raw or cooked - they are nutritious in all forms. Vitamin B6 is important as it forms a sheath of protein around myelin. Hence, keeping an adequate amount of pyridoxine is essential.

What are the Benefits Of Vitamin B6?

There are several benefits of Vitamin B6.

Vitamin B6 Helps In Keeping Your Heart Healthy
One of the 21 amino acids in your body is called homocysteine. If the levels of homocysteine are elevated, this will result in problems in the heart. [97]Pyridoxine ensures that there is not an extra accumulation of this amino acid in your body. This helps to keep your heart healthy.

Vitamin B6 Helps In Reducing The Morning Sickness
Pyridoxine has been used for a long time in the treatment of morning sickness and nausea that happens during pregnancy. In fact, Vitamin B6 is an active ingredient in some common medications that are used to treat morning sickness too.

Though it has not been concluded the reason it helps to do so, it is believed that a sufficient amount of Vitamin B6 is essential for a healthy pregnancy.

If you experience severe morning sickness, you can always have a conversation with your doctor regarding this and have the vitamin B6 supplements if the doctor prescribes them.

---

[97]*Homocysteine Test: MedlinePlus Lab Test Information.* (2018). Medlineplus.gov. https://medlineplus.gov/lab-tests/homocysteine-test/

If you're interested in taking B6 for morning sickness, speak with your doctor before starting any supplements.

Vitamin B6 Helps Strengthen The Immune System Of The Body
Vitamin B6 aids the immune system by regulating chemical reactions. This helps to keep your body guarded against different types of infection. People with a low pyridoxine level will showcase a poor immune response. [98]

Vitamin B6 Helps In The Betterment Of The Function Of The Brain
Many studies suggest that Vitamin B6 plays an essential role in the health of the brain, and it is also linked with the prevention of Alzheimer's disease.

Vitamin B6 Helps To Lower The Risk Of Cancer
As per some research, it has been observed that when there is an adequate amount of Vitamin B6 in the blood, it helps decrease the risk of cancer. [99] If you are a patient with cancer, ingestion of Vitamin B6 has been linked with the slower growth of the tumor.

Vitamin B6 Helps In The Betterment Of Mood
Vitamin B6, or pyridoxine, aids the body in making serotonin. [100] Serotonin is a hormone that helps in the elevation of your mood and keeps you content. According to some studies, lower levels of Vitamin B6 were linked to depression.

---

[98] Qian, B., Shen, S., Zhang, J., & Jing, P. (2017). Effects of Vitamin B6 Deficiency on the Composition and Functional Potential of T Cell Populations. *Journal of Immunology Research, 2017.* https://doi.org/10.1155/2017/2197975

[99] National Institutes of Health. (2017). *Office of Dietary Supplements - Vitamin B6.* Nih.gov. https://ods.od.nih.gov/factsheets/vitaminB6-healthprofessional/

[100] *9 Health Benefits of Vitamin B6 (Pyridoxine).* (2018, October 1). Healthline. https://www.healthline.com/nutrition/vitamin-b6-benefits#TOC_TITLE_HDR_2

Vitamin B6 Helps In Dealing With The Effects Of PMS

It has been seen in many cases that taking supplements of Vitamin B6 has resulted in helping with the effects of premenstrual syndrome. Some of the symptoms it helps in easing are depression, anxiety, and breast tenderness.

Importance of Vitamin B7 (Biotin)

What is Vitamin B7?

Vitamin B7 is also commonly known as biotin or vitamin H.[101] It is one of the vitamins from the B-complex too. Biotin is a vitamin that is water-soluble, which means it can be dissolved easily in water. This vitamin is crucial for the body as it helps in the metabolism of carbohydrates, proteins, and fats.

The water-soluble vitamins are not stored in the body and are excreted by the process of urine. Hence we need to make sure that there is daily consumption of this vitamin. Vitamin B7 is unable to be synthesized by the cells of the body, but t can be synthesized by some specific bacteria that are present in the body of humans. You can also get an adequate supply of Vitamin B7 through the foods that you consume.

Biotin is widely used to promote the growth of cells. People use biotin supplements in order to make their nails and hair strong. Other than Vitamin B7, and Biotin, it is called Vitamin H due to the German words "Haut" and "Haar," which means skin and hair.

If you have insufficient levels of Vitamin B7, it can affect your nails, hair, nervous system, and skin. You can make sure that you eat food that has biotin in them, like egg yolk, avocado, biotin-rich vegetables, liver, etc. You can also get Vitamin B7 prescribed by your health care adviser.

---

[101] *Biotin (Vitamin B7): Uses, sources, and health benefits.* (2017, October 18). Www.medicalnewstoday.com.
https://www.medicalnewstoday.com/articles/287720

What Natural Sources Can You Get Vitamin B7 From?

Vitamin B7 is essential for your body as it helps the body to convert the food that you ingest into a form of energy. [102]Being a water-soluble vitamin in nature, it is excreted out of the body as urine rather than stored. Hence, you need to ensure that the daily consumption of this vitamin is done in order to have sufficient levels of it.

You can have Vitamin B7 as a supplement or from a diet that is rich in biotin.

Some natural sources of Vitamin B7 are mentioned below.

Egg Yolk

Eating an egg is a nutritious option, especially when it comes to biotin. A yolk of an egg is recognized as a good biotin source. [103]If you eat an entire cooked egg, you will be getting around ten mcg of biotin from it; this makes up around 33% of the required biotin levels in the body. If you eat eggs in raw form, you will not be able to get the complete nutritious benefits of it. This is because of the presence of a protein in the raw egg named dietary avidin - this protein creates a bond with biotin that creates difficulty in absorption by the body. When you cook the egg, the protein and the biotin are separated, which provides the digestive tract with the chance to absorb the vitamin; other than that, cooking the eggs also aids in decreasing the risk of Salmonella poisoning.

Eggs are a good source of B-complex vitamins, phosphorus, protein, and iron. Rather than the white part, the yolk contains a richer level of biotin in it.

---

[102] *Health Benefits of Biotin: What Does the Science Say?* (2015). Healthline. https://www.healthline.com/health/the-benefits-of-biotin

[103] *9 biotin-rich foods to add to your diet.* (2019, December 6). Www.medicalnewstoday.com. https://www.medicalnewstoday.com/articles/320222

You can eat the eggs in any form you like; they can be scrambled, boiled, fried, or poached.

Liver

Cooked chicken liver is a rich option for your biotin intake.[104] If you consume three ounces of chicken liver, it will give you 138 mcg of biotin. This is 460% of the total required amount by the body.

If you consume cooked beef liver, you can consume good levels of biotin. This is due to the fact that whatever little biotin is present in the body is stacked in the liver. If you consume three ounces of beef liver, it will provide you with 31 mcg of biotin! This is a sufficient amount of biotin in your body and reaches 103% of the required amount of biotin levels. If you eat liver, it can help in giving a boost to your biotin levels in the body. The beef liver also contains iron and can aid in getting your iron levels sorted too.

Other than beef liver, you can also consume kidneys for biotin consumption.

Avocado

If you consume about 100 g of avocados, they will contain 3.2 - 10 mcg of biotin in it. Avocados are also a good source of Vitamin E and are considered good for the health of the skin. [105]You can eat the avocados in any form that you like; they can be put on toast or can be used raw; they can also be used in salads, burritos, and even guacamole.

---

[104] *9 biotin-rich foods to add to your diet*. (2019, December 6). Www.medicalnewstoday.com. https://www.medicalnewstoday.com/articles/320222

[105] Kubala, J. (2021, November 26). *7 Benefits of Eating Avocados, According to a Dietitian*. Healthline. https://www.healthline.com/nutrition/avocado-nutrition

Salmon

While being enriched with Omega-3 fats, Salmon also consists of Vitamin B7. If you eat three ounces of cooked Salmon, it can provide you with five mcg of Vitamin B7. It is very beneficial for the health of your hair and protects your hair from facing an extreme hair fall.

Nuts & Seeds

Different nuts and seeds contain different levels of biotin in it. Biotin is present in peanuts, pecans, almonds, walnuts, and sunflower seeds. [106]

Along with biotin, nuts and seeds also contain unsaturated fat, proteins, and fiber. You can incorporate them into your meals in multiple ways, like mixing them up with salads, stir-frying them with pasta, making butter consisting of nuts and seeds, or just eating a handful of raw nuts.

Legumes

Consuming legumes is very good for health as they are rich in fiber, protein as well as many other micronutrients too. [107]

Legumes can be utilized as a base for salads or can be stir-fried too.

Sweet Potatoes

Sweet potatoes are stacked with biotin, fibers, minerals, minerals, etc. Where vegetables are concerned, sweet potatoes take the lead in being the best source of biotin.

---

[106] *9 biotin-rich foods to add to your diet.* (2019, December 6). Www.medicalnewstoday.com.
https://www.medicalnewstoday.com/articles/320222

[107] *Legumes: Good or Bad?* (2016). Healthline.
https://www.healthline.com/nutrition/legumes-good-or-bad

When you consume 125 g of sweet potatoes in cooked forms, you can get around 2.4 mcg of biotin. This makes up around 8% of the required dietary allowance of biotin levels.

You can use baked potatoes by microwaving them or baking them. You can also give it a bit of a twist and peel them, put them for boiling, then get to mashing them up - and eat it up.

Yeast

When it comes to yeast, nutritional yeast and brewer's yeast both serve as good sources of Vitamin B7. [108]The level of biotin depends on the brand of the yeast. The inactive yeast that is used to give a nutty or cheesy flavor to the food is nutritional yeast. Brewer's yeast is an active yeast that is used in the making of bread and beer.

21 mcg of Vitamin B7 is present in two tablespoons of nutritional yeast, which makes up 69% of the requirement.

While a 2.25 teaspoon of active yeast contains 1.4 much Vitamin B7, which makes up 5% of the total requirement of biotin per day.

What are the Benefits of Vitamin B7?

The consumption of Vitamin B7 leads to many benefits. You need a regular intake of this essential vitamin to keep a sufficient amount of it in the body. Vitamin B7 is very important as it helps in many functions.

Vitamin B7 Helps in A Stable Pregnancy

To ensure that the baby is healthy during pregnancy, biotin is often prescribed to pregnant ladies. [109]It is also added to folic acid. The doctor should prescribe it as high doses of Vitamin B7 can

---

[108] *The Top 10 Biotin-Rich Foods.* (2020, July 24). Healthline. https://www.healthline.com/nutrition/biotin-rich-foods

[109] *Pregnancy B Vitamins: How Important Are They?* (2015, September 3). Healthline. https://www.healthline.com/health/pregnancy/b-vitamins

also prove to be dangerous for the baby. Due to this, you should not use it without getting a recommendation from your doctor.

Vitamin B7 Helps in Managing Diabetes
According to many studies, Vitamin B7 also helps to decrease the level of blood glucose in people suffering from type 1 or type 2 diabetes. [110]According to scientists, Vitamin B7 aids in the stimulation of the pancreas that secretes insulin; this helps in decreasing blood glucose levels.

In patients with Type 1 diabetes, biotin helps to aid in glycemic control. Studies are in the process of proving this benefit.

Vitamin B7 Helps in The Improvement of Nails, Hair, And Skin
According to studies, the intake of biotin can help in the improvement of the nails, hair, and skin. It is observed that an adequate quantity of biotin results in increasing the strength of the nails and can also thicken them. Due to the biotin levels, the breakage is reduced too.

Due to Vitamin B7, the health of the skin is improved too. It helps to add glow to the skin and also helps in strengthening the hair.

Vitamin B7 Helps to Regulate the Metabolic System
Vitamin B7 is important in carrying out the metabolism of carbohydrates, protein, and fats in an efficient manner. [111]It helps support carboxylase enzymes also. These enzymes are important because they help in the synthesis of fatty acids, amino acids valine, and isoleucine, and also help in the process of gluconeogenesis.

---

[110] *Biotin (Vitamin B7): Uses, sources, and health benefits.* (2017, October 18). Www.medicalnewstoday.com. https://www.medicalnewstoday.com/articles/287720

[111] *Vitamin B7/Biotin: Functions, Food Sources, Deficiencies and Toxicity.* (n.d.). Netmeds. https://www.netmeds.com/health-library/post/vitamin-b7-functions-food-sources-deficiencies-and-toxicity

Vitamin B7 Promotes the Function of the Brain

The B7 Vitamin of the B-complex is also important as it helps in promoting the function of the brain in a healthy manner. Due to biotin, the management of many neurological symptoms is managed. This includes the management of neuropathy as well as when the nerve undergoes damage.

Importance of Vitamin B9 (Folate)

What is Vitamin B9?

Vitamin B9 is also called folate. This vitamin is also a part of B-complex vitamins, and it has water-soluble properties. This means that it can easily dissolve in water. This vitamin naturally occurs in many foods; other than that, you can also take supplements of this vitamin - the supplements you can intake will be under the name of folic acid.

You can absorb folic acid more efficiently in your body than absorption through natural food sources.[112]

When our body absorbs Vitamin B9 from natural sources, it absorbs 50% of it, while if we compare it with folic acid supplements, the absorption level increases to 85%. The folate is very important.

Folate is very important as it helps produce RNA and DNA.[113] This aids in the metabolism of protein. It is also essential because of its role in breaking down amino acids with homocysteine. If the homocysteine is present in high amounts, it can result in toxic effects in the body. Other than that, for the production of healthy red blood cells, folate is needed too. Folate is a very important vitamin and is essential during the growing phase, like pregnancy and fetus development. During pregnancy, folic acid is recommended by doctors mainly as it helps to decrease the risk of congenital disabilities linked with neural tubes; the neural tube is the structure that helps in the formation of the brain and spinal cord, and the defect in this neural tubes can be decreased due to

---

[112] Harvard T.H. Chan. (2012, September 18). *Folate (Folic Acid) – Vitamin B9*. The Nutrition Source. https://www.hsph.harvard.edu/nutritionsource/folic-acid/

[113] Harvard T.H. Chan. (2012, September 18). *Folate (Folic Acid) – Vitamin B9*. The Nutrition Source. https://www.hsph.harvard.edu/nutritionsource/folic-acid/

the entail of folic acid. It helps decrease the risk of spina bifida and cleft lip and protects the brain from any damage.

Many people suffer from a low level of folic acid. Some causes of folic acid deficiency are inflammatory bowel disease (IBD), alcoholism, and celiac disease. The levels of folic acid can also be decreased due to the effects of some medications, and the deficiency of folic acid can also result in problems like the effect on growth and inflammation in the tongue. In gingivitis, some people also experience a loss of appetite or problems breathing. Other than that, it also causes diarrhea, the inability to remember things at times, an irritated mood can also occur, and people may even experience mental sluggishness.

In the United States of America, folic acid is being added to many foods like cereal and bread; due to this, an observation has been made on the dramatic decrease of neural tube defects.

What Natural Sources Can You Get Vitamin B9 From?

Vitamin B9 is important for the body as it helps in the diction of healthy cells of the body and helps promote the growth of the fetus in a proper way. [114] This helps to decrease the chances of defects in the fetus.

Vitamin B9 can be taken through natural foods, folic acid supplements, and fortified foods. Some natural sources of Vitamin B9 are mentioned below.

---

[114] Harvard T.H. Chan. (2012, September 18). *Folate (Folic Acid) – Vitamin B9*. The Nutrition Source. https://www.hsph.harvard.edu/nutritionsource/folic-acid/

Legumes

Legumes include the seeds or fruits of plants belonging to the Plant Kingdom's Fabaceae family. These include peas, beans, and also lentils. All the different legumes are known to be having different amounts of folate in them, but they are considered a really good source of Vitamin B9.[115]

If you cook 1 cup of kidney beans, it will contain around 131 mcg of folate, making up about 33% of the required daily value in the body. Comparatively, if you decide to cook 1 cup of lentils, you will be getting around 358 mcg of folate. This will give you 90% of the required daily value of folate.

Seeds And Nuts

If you are a person who is not very fond of nuts or seeds, you should think about some important things that you are going to miss out on. When we talk about seeds and nuts, they contain a good value of protein and are also enriched with fiber, and it also contains minerals required by the human body.

If you make it a habit to eat seeds and nuts on a regular basis, this can help you up to your folate levels. We can see a little variation in the amount of folate that is present in nuts and seeds. If we consider 1 oz of walnuts, they will give you about 28 mcg of folate; this will make up about 7% of the required value for the day. If you consume 1 oz of flax seeds, this will provide you with 24 mcg of folate, which will make up about 6% of the total required value of the human body.

---

[115] Link, R. (2018, May 22). *15 Healthy Foods That Are High in Folate (Folic Acid)*. Healthline; Healthline Media.
https://www.healthline.com/nutrition/foods-high-in-folate-folic-acid

Broccoli

Broccoli is known in the world due to its health-promoting properties, and the addition of it to your diet can help in the consumption of a wide variety of minerals as well as vitamins.[116]

If you consume 1 cup of broccoli, this would mean that you have consumed around 57 mcg of folate, which would make up about 14% of the required allowance for the day. When you eat the cooked form of broccoli, it helps you in achieving a larger quantity of folate that would increase to 84 mcg for half a cup, and this would make up about 21% of the required dietary allowance.

Asparagus

If you like to eat asparagus, you would be delighted to know that it contains a good amount of many minerals and vitamins that include Vitamin B9. [117]

If you consume half a cup of asparagus that is in cooked form, you will be able to get 134 mcg of folate through it. This will make up around 34% of the required value for one day.

What are the Benefits of Vitamin B9?

If you talk about folic acid or folate, we can also find them in the form of supplements. While we can observe that folate and folic acid are used in the same condition, they have two different processes for metabolism, and this can cause affect your health.

---

[116] *Broccoli: Health benefits, nutrition, and tips*. (2020, January 9). www.medicalnewstoday.com.
https://www.medicalnewstoday.com/articles/266765
[117] Coyle, D. (2018, April 4). *Top 7 Health Benefits of Asparagus*. Healthline. https://www.healthline.com/nutrition/asparagus-benefits

We have mentioned the benefits of Vitamin B9 below:

Vitamin B9 Helps In the Treatment of Mental Health Conditions

Vitamin B9 is essential in the development of neurotransmitters in the brain.[118] These are the chemicals of the brain, and if the development of neurotransmitters ceases, it can cause problems in the brain. People who did not have adequate levels of folate in their bodies were linked with mental problems like schizophrenia, depression, etc. According to a study, people with depression showcased reduced amounts of folate.

Vitamin B9 Helps In a Healthy Pregnancy

It is imperative to aid in a healthy pregnancy. Regarding birth defects, folic acid is the key to reducing their risk in newborns. [119]If folic acid is consumed during pregnancy, this will help in a safe pregnancy with lesser risks. Other than this, they are also important in pregnancy as they help in the development of the fetus and also aid in lowering the chance of complications in pregnancy like preeclampsia.

Vitamin B9 Reduces the Risk of a Heart Attack

If you use supplements of folate or folic acid, this can help decrease the risk of a heart attack. Heart attacks are common occurrences due to the high presence of an amino acid named homocysteine. Folate helps decrease this risk by breaking down the homocysteine in the body so that there aren't high levels of it.

---

[118] McGarel C, Pentieva K, Strain JJ, McNulty H. Emerging roles for folate and related B-vitamins in brain health across the lifecycle. Proc Nutr Soc. 2015 Feb;74(1):46-55. doi: 10.1017/S0029665114001554. Epub 2014 Nov 5. PMID: 25371067.

[119] CDC. (2020, January 2). Folic Acid Helps Prevent Some Birth Defects. Centers for Disease Control and Prevention.
https://www.cdc.gov/ncbddd/folicacid/features/folic-acid-helps-prevent-some-birth-defects.html

Importance of Vitamin B12 (Cobalamin)

What is Vitamin B12?

Vitamin B12 is also known as Cobalamin. It is an essential component that your body requires to carry out the synthesis of DNA, the production of energy, and also to carry out the functions of the central nervous system. [120]

Vitamin B12 is found in a wide variety of food, but still, it is seen that the deficiency of vitamin B12 is prevalent. This happens mainly because of limited intake of foods that have vitamin B12, medical conditions, malabsorption, or the usage of medications that deplete the levels of Vitamin B12.

According to a study, around 20% of the people who exceed the age of 60 in the United Kingdom and the United States of America are said to have a deficiency of Vitamin B12. While it is common in the elderly, it does not mean it can not occur in the younger. As the age grows, the body finds it harder to absorb Vitamin B12; hence this deficiency occurs in the body.

If you think you have a deficiency of Vitamin B12, you can go to your healthcare advisor and discuss your symptoms, and they can recommend the appropriate tests for your symptoms.

Vitamin B12 is a vitamin of the B-complex and is water-soluble in nature. [121] It can dissolve in water. Being water-soluble in nature, it is not stored in the body, so you should intake sufficient levels of Vitamin B12 regularly so that you have

---

[120] Calderón-Ospina, C. A., & Nava-Mesa, M. O. (2019). B Vitamins in the nervous system: Current knowledge of the biochemical modes of action and synergies of thiamine, pyridoxine, and cobalamin. *CNS Neuroscience & Therapeutics*, 26(1), 5–13. https://doi.org/10.1111/cns.13207

[121] Lykstad, J., & Sharma, S. (2022). *Biochemistry, Water Soluble Vitamins*. PubMed; StatPearls Publishing.
https://www.ncbi.nlm.nih.gov/books/NBK538510

adequate levels of this Vitamin. Vitamin B12 is excreted out of the body through the process of urination.

This Vitamin can be found in many foods; for instance, it can be found in dairy, fish, and meat and can also be taken as a supplement. The active form in which Vitamin B12 occurs is called Methylcobalamin. There is one form known as cyanocobalamin that is supposed to be activated by the body. This is mainly found in supplements as well.

What Natural Sources Can You Get Vitamin B12 From?

It is important to consume sufficient levels of Vitamin B12. This is because they are perfect for your health. It can be made sure that you have sufficient levels of vitamin B12 through food sources. But, if people consume only plant-based meals, they would have to eat foods fortified with B12 or B12 supplements to maintain the levels properly. Vitamin B12 is very important for the synthesis of DNA, functions of the brain, and also the formation of red blood cells. [122]Hence, we need to make sure that we do not go through a deficiency of Vitamin B12. Due to its functions, a person with a deficiency of Vitamin B12 can suffer from psychiatric and anemic symptoms.

You can get Vitamin B12 from many food sources. These food sources include the following:

Liver and Kidneys
Consuming an animal's cooked kidneys and liver helps us stack on Vitamin B12 levels.[123] The different animals offer

---

[122] Felman, A. (2017, November 28). *Vitamin B-12: Functions, deficiency, and sources*. Www.medicalnewstoday.com.
https://www.medicalnewstoday.com/articles/219822

[123] Semeco, A. (2018, May 3). *Top 12 Foods That Are High in Vitamin B12*. Healthline; Healthline Media. https://www.healthline.com/nutrition/vitamin-b12-foods

different levels of Vitamin B12, but lambs are considered the best source of Cobalamin. Consuming a hundred grams of the cooked liver of lamb provides 3.571% of the recommended levels of this Vitamin. This is the reason that the lamb liver takes the lead on the levels of Vitamin B12. The liver of beef or veal is close behind and offers 3.000% of the recommended value of Vitamin B12. Along with Vitamin B12, the liver of the lamb is also packed with other nutrients like selenium, vitamin A, etc.

Milk

When it comes to dairy, milk takes the lead in Vitamin B12 levels. If you can not drink milk, you can hunt for alternatives with Vitamin B12 on the labels. It can be almond milk, cashew milk, oat milk, soy milk, etc.

Shellfish

When we talk about shellfish, clams are enriched with many nutrients and vitamin B12. It [124]is enriched with proteins and also has Vitamin B12 in it. If you consume 190 grams of clams, you can get 7000% of the RDV. They also have iron in them as well as antioxidants. The best way to consume is to have the broth of clams by boiling them - it is rich in vitamin B12. You can also consume the canned clam broth - 3.5 ounces contains 112-588% of the recommended value of Vitamin B12.

Fortified Cereals

Being a vegetarian, you can get your vitamin B12 levels sorted by eating fortified cereals. You can be smart with the other benefits and get a cereal that has decreased amount of sugar and increased amounts of whole grains and fiber. These can help you elevate the levels of Vitamin B12 in your body.

---

[124] Ibid.

Fish

When it comes to fish, 100 grams of Sardines contain 8.94 mcg of Vitamin B12[125]. These are soft-boned fishes that are mainly sold in canned form. They can be canned in oil, water, or sauces, and if you wish, you can also buy them fresh; sardines are stacked with a variety of nutrients and is considered a very nutritious and important fish. If we consume one cup of sardines, we can get 554% of the recommended dietary values of Vitamin B12.

Other than that, Sardines also contain omega-3 fatty acids that help in the improvement of the heart as well as aid in reducing inflammation.

Other than Sardines, Tuna, Salmon, and Trout also contain certain levels of Vitamin B12.

Eggs

If you are consuming eggs for the purpose of Vitamin B12, you need to focus on the egg yolks more than the white part.[126] They contain more Vitamin B12 than egg whites. However, you can eat the entire eggs to increase the level of Vitamin B12.

Yogurt

Eating low-fat Greek yogurt provides you with a Vitamin B12 increment and is accepted as a healthy option for the intake of Vitamin B12. Eating full-fat and plain yogurt can even raise vitamin B12 levels as the Vitamin can be readily absorbed in dairy.

What are the Benefits of Vitamin B12?

---

[125] *Are sardines good for you? Nutritional benefits and more.* (2020, November 30). Www.medicalnewstoday.com.
https://www.medicalnewstoday.com/articles/are-sardines-good-for-you

[126] Semeco, A. (2018, May 3). *Top 12 Foods That Are High in Vitamin B12*. Healthline; Healthline Media. https://www.healthline.com/nutrition/vitamin-b12-foods

Vitamin B12 has many benefits for the human body. It actively offers support to the nerve cells of the body and also helps boost the production of red blood cells. [127] The synthesis of DNA is also made possible due to Vitamin B12. Some of the benefits of Cobalamin are mentioned below.

Vitamin B12 Help In Supporting The Skin, Nails, And Hair

With the help of Vitamin B12, the production of new cells is done. Due to this, the body is able to have healthy skin, nails, and also hair. Studies have shown that having a deficiency in vitamin B12 in the body can result in the discoloration of nails, changes in the hair, hyperpigmentation of the skin, vitiligo, and uneven angular stomatitis. [128] In vitiligo, a person faces a fading of skin color, and it happens in patches. In angular stomatitis, the mouth corners can be seen to have inflammation and cracked skin.

Improving the levels of Vitamin B12 in the body has improved the symptoms of the nails, hair, and skin.

Vitamin B12 Helps in Keeping the Heart Healthy

If there is a high level of particular amino acid, the name homocysteine, in the blood, it can disrupt the health of the heart. [129]With the deficiency of vitamin B12, the homocysteine levels are observed to elevate. This helps in increasing the risk of heart disease.

If you have sufficient levels of Vitamin B12 in your body, it is observed that the homocysteine levels decrease along with the risk

---

[127] Felman, A. (2017, November 28). *Vitamin B-12: Functions, deficiency, and sources*.www.medicalnewstoday.com.https://www.medicalnewstoday.com/articles/219822

[128] Kannan, R., & Ng, M. J. M. (2008). Cutaneous lesions and vitamin B12 deficiency: an often-forgotten link. Canadian Family Physician Medecin de Famille Canadien, 54(4), 529 532. https://www.ncbi.nlm.nih.gov/pmc/articles/PMC2294086/

[129] *Homocysteine: Levels, Tests, High Homocysteine Levels*. (n.d.). Cleveland Clinic. https://my.clevelandclinic.org/health/articles/21527-homocysteine

of heart disease. This is based purely on studies, and no scientific evidence has yet been formed on it.

Vitamin B12 Is Linked To the Loss of Neurons in the Brain
When you have low levels of Vitamin B12, you can often go through a loss of memory. It usually occurs in people who reach old age. Vitamin B12 is very important in preventing the atrophy of the brain, which can later result in dementia or memory loss. [130]

During one study, it was observed that the levels of Vitamin B12 combined with omega-3 tended to decrease the decline in mental levels. Other than that, it was observed that when the levels of Vitamin B12 were low, the people showed low memory performance too. Hence, Vitamin B12 is considered important, and supplements of it are suggested if it is not taken in its natural forms.

---

[130] Rabensteiner, J., Hofer, E., Fauler, G., Fritz-Petrin, E., Benke, T., Dal-Bianco, P., Ransmayr, G., Schmidt, R., & Herrmann, M. (2020). The impact of folate and vitamin B12 status on cognitive function and brain atrophy in healthy elderly and demented Austrians, a retrospective cohort study. *Aging, 12*(15), 15478–15491. https://doi.org/10.18632/aging.103714

Vitamin B12 Is Linked With the Improvement in Depression and Can Also Help Elevate the Mood

It is observed that adequate levels of Vitamin B12 can help in the improvement of mood as well as depression. Cobalamin is an essential vitamin that helps synthesize and metabolize serotonin. This chemical is very important for the proper regulation of mood.

Hence, low levels of Vitamin B12 may end up in a decrease in serotonin, which can result in depression and a bad mood. [131] It was observed that the people who consumed Vitamin B12 had good levels of improved mood compared to those with lower levels of Vitamin B12.

Also, it was seen that the deficiency of Cobalamin was closely linked to double the risk of severe depression. People suffering from Major Depressive Disorder have been seen to be recovered completely with the appropriate levels of Vitamin B12.

This data is not scientifically backed, even though it portrays many cases where it serves as a mood booster.

Vitamin B12 Helps In Producing Red Blood Cells (RBCs) In The Human Body

Vitamin B12 is essential for the body as it helps in the formation of red blood cells (RBCs). If [132]the body does not have a significant amount of vitamin B12 in the body, it will result in a reduction in the formation of red blood cells, and also, there can be hindrances in the proper formation of red blood cells.

---

[131] Vitamin B-12 Deficiency and Depression: What's the Link? (2017, January 12). Healthline. https://www.healthline.com/health/depression/b12-and-depression

[132] *Vitamin B12 deficiency anemia: MedlinePlus Medical Encyclopedia.* (n.d.). Medlineplus.gov. https://medlineplus.gov/ency/article/000574.html

If you study a healthy red blood cell, it will be perfectly round in shape. When the body goes through a deficiency in vitamin B12, the red blood cells become oval in shape.

Due to the oval shape, the red blood cells undergo problems transporting from the bone marrow into the bloodstream at the usual rate - and because of this, megaloblastic anemia can be caused[133]. Due to anemia, the body does not have the required red blood cells to transport oxygen to all organs in an orderly manner. This results in weakness and fatigue in the human body.

Vitamin B12 Can Help In the Prevention of Birth Defects
According to studies, it is seen that the brain of the fetus requires vitamin B12 from the mother to develop in a proper manner. This is considered essential in order to have a healthy pregnancy.

If you consume enough amount of Vitamin B12 in the initial stages of pregnancy, it can help in reducing the risk of birth defects like neural tube defects. If the mother does not have sufficient Vitamin B12 in her diet, it can also result in a miscarriage or premature birth. This is not proven yet, rather than observed through studies.

Vitamin B12 Helps in Supporting the Health of the Bone
If your body has adequate levels of B12, it can help in supporting the health of your bone. [134]A study that included 2,500 people showcased that the people who had lower levels of vitamin B12 also indicated a lower bone density than usual.

Bones that have a reduced mineral density can become fragile and delicate as time passes, and they can also hold an increased

---

[133] Anis Hariz, & Bhattacharya, P. T. (2019, January 23). Megaloblastic Anemia. Nih.gov; StatPearls Publishing. https://www.ncbi.nlm.nih.gov/books/NBK537254/

[134] Berkheiser, K. (2018, June 14). 9 Health Benefits of Vitamin B12, Based on Science. Healthline; Healthline Media. https://www.healthline.com/nutrition/vitamin-b12-benefits

risk for osteoporosis. There is a link between vitamin B12 levels and bone health, and this is seen more in women.

Importance of Vitamin C (Ascorbic Acid)

What is Vitamin C?

Vitamin C is also called Ascorbic Acid and is a very important vitamin. It should be consumed in the form of vegetables and fruits, especially citrus ones.

Vitamin C is essential for a strong immune system.[135] According to the experts, rather than taking supplements for Vitamin C, it is best to take adequate amounts of it through your diet.

Make a habit of drinking freshly squeezed orange juice, as it can help boost the levels of Vitamin C in your body. [136]

This Vitamin is also water-soluble. Regular consumption of Vitamin C is important for maintaining healthy levels in the body. It can be eaten in natural forms or added to food. People also consume supplements of these vitamins.

---

[135] *How Vitamin C Supports a Healthy Immune System.* (2019). Eatright.org. https://www.eatright.org/food/vitamins-and-supplements/types-of-vitamins-and-nutrients/how-vitamin-c-supports-a-healthy-immune-system

[136] Link, R. (2019, February 12). *5 Surprising Health Benefits of Orange Juice.* Healthline; Healthline Media. https://www.healthline.com/nutrition/orange-juice-benefits

What Natural Sources Can You Get Vitamin C From?

You can get Vitamin C from many natural sources. Some of them are mentioned below:

Guavas
This delicious fruit is pink-fleshed and is found in Mexico and South America, along with other places. When you consume one, you can get 125 mg of vitamin C through it, which makes up 138% of the recommended dietary value.

Oranges
A single, medium-sized orange will give you 83 mg of vitamin C, which constitutes 92% of the required dietary value. It is very commonly used to boost natural levels in the body organically.

Plums
The plums - especially Kakadu plums that are native to Australia contain Vitamin C, which is 100 times more than in oranges. In 100gms of these plums, you can get 2,907 mg of vitamin C. Besides Ascorbic acid, the Kakadu plums are also rich in Vitamin E, potassium, and lutein. [137]

Rose Hip
It is a sweet and tangy fruit that is small in size and is derived from the rose plant. This fruit is stacked with Vitamin C. Consuming 100 g of this fruit can give you 426 mg of Vitamin C, which would make up around 473% of the recommended dietary value.

---

[137] Which Foods Are High In Vitamin C – Health Insurance Blog By Reliance General. (n.d.). Www.reliancegeneral.co.in. Retrieved November 11, 2022, from https://www.reliancegeneral.co.in/Insurance/Knowledge-Center/Blogs/List-Of-Foods-That-Are-High-In-Vitamin-C.aspx

Cherries

Consuming 49 g of acerola cherries is known to give around 825 mg of Vitamin C, which is about 916% of the recommended dietary levels. Along with this, these cherries are also stacked with polyphenols. Due to the Vitamin C present in them, cherries are considered to have antioxidant properties.

Chilli Peppers

If you are a person who loves spicy things, you would be surprised to know that a single chili pepper has 109 mg of vitamin C in it[138]; this would make up 121% of the recommended dietary levels in the body. Research is still going on to fully link the health benefits of chili peppers to the body.

Blackcurrants

Consuming half a cup of blackcurrants will give you around 102 mg of vitamin C. [139] This will make up 113% of the Recommended Dietary Values. The antioxidant flavonoids present in it help to provide the dark and rich color that the blackcurrants possess.

---

[138] Did you know that hot chilli peppers have more Vitamin C than oranges? Health benefits of the popular spice. (n.d.). Www.timesnownews.com. Retrieved November 11, 2022, from https://www.timesnownews.com/health/article/did-you-know-that-hot-chilli-peppers-have-more-vitamin-c-than-oranges-health-benefits-of-the-popular-spice/654351

[139] Hill, C. (2018). *20 Foods That Are High in Vitamin C*. Healthline. https://www.healthline.com/nutrition/vitamin-c-foods

What are the Benefits of Vitamin C?

Vitamin C has several benefits. Some of them are mentioned below:

Vitamin C Helps In Decreasing The Risk Of Chronic Disease
Vitamin C is a strong antioxidant that strengthens the body and boosts the immune system. It does that by protecting cells from free radicals.

Chronic diseases are often caused by oxidative stress due to the accumulation of free radicals.

With enough vitamin C, you can have sufficient antioxidants in the body that help battle inflammation and strengthen natural defenses.

Vitamin C Manages High Blood Pressure
Vitamin C helps manage high blood pressure, thus keeping the heart healthy. [140]High blood pressure can cause a stroke and other heart diseases.

According to studies, Vitamin C lowers blood pressure and relaxes the blood vessels.

Vitamin C Prevents Iron Deficiency
Iron is a very important nutrient in the body that is used in making red blood cells.[141] Vitamin C allows our body to absorb iron easily.

If a person has low levels of iron, they can consider talking to their healthcare advisor about Vitamin C intake to manage it.

---

[140] *Big Doses of Vitamin C May Lower Blood Pressure - 04/18/2012.* (n.d.). Www.hopkinsmedicine.org.
https://www.hopkinsmedicine.org/news/media/releases/big_doses_of_vitamin_c_may_lower_blood_pressure

[141] *Iron in diet: MedlinePlus Medical Encyclopedia.* (2019). Medlineplus.gov. https://medlineplus.gov/ency/article/002422.ht

Vitamin C Helps in Boosting the Immunity of the Body

Vitamin C helps in boosting immunity of the body by aiding in the production of white blood cells. It helps produce phagocytes and lymphocytes that help to protect the body against infection in the body.

Besides the production, it also helps the White blood cells function effectively and protects them from free radicals.

Vitamin C Helps in Lowering the Risk of Heart Disease

Vitamin C is known to be excellent in battling high blood pressure and dealing with high levels of LDL and low levels of HDL.[142]

Due to this, a reduction can be seen in the risk of heart disease. According to a study that had 293,172 people, it was seen that people who took 700 mg of Vitamin C regularly had a 25% lesser risk of heart disease than those who did not consume Vitamin C.

However, it is not scientifically proven as yet.

---

[142] Jacques, P. F. (1992). Effects of vitamin C on high-density lipoprotein cholesterol and blood pressure. *Journal of the American College of Nutrition, 11*(2), 139–144. https://pubmed.ncbi.nlm.nih.gov/1578088/

Importance of Vitamin D (Calciferol)

What is Vitamin D?

Vitamin D is also called calciferol. It works as two things - a vitamin and also a hormone. [143]

Unlike the B-complex vitamins, this one is fat-soluble in nature. This vitamin is essential for the body as it aids in the absorption of phosphorus and calcium - these are both very important to building bone. According to studies, it is seen that adequate amounts of Vitamin D can help in the reduction of the growth of cancer. It also helps in controlling infections and works to decrease the effects of inflammation. It has been researched that Vitamin D receptors are found in many different body organs and tissues. This indicates that this paves the way for more functions done by this particular vitamin.

There are not many foods that contain Vitamin D naturally. Some foods are also fortified with this important vitamin. Most people get their dose of Vitamin D through supplements as it is hard to get enough Vitamin D from food. You can find Vitamin D supplements in two main forms; one is known as Vitamin D3 (known as Cholecalciferol), and the other one is known as Vitamin D2 (known as pre-Vitamin D or ergocalciferol). These two forms of vitamin D also occur naturally through the UVB rays of the sun - this is the reason why it is nicknamed "The Sunshine Vitamin". D2 is not produced in the human body. [144] Instead, it's produced in fungi and plants. Vitamin D3 is procured in humans and animals. People often have reduced doses of vitamin D in winter because of the limited sunlight that occurs in winter. Also, if

---

[143] Vitamin D | You and Your Hormones from the Society for Endocrinology. (n.d.). Www.yourhormones.info. https://www.yourhormones.info/hormones/vitamin-d/

[144] *Vitamin D Metabolism and Function.* (2015, January 6). ALPCO. https://www.alpco.com/vitamin-d-metabolism-func

someone does not go out in the sun a lot, they can suffer from a deficiency of Vitamin D.

What Natural Sources Can You Get Vitamin D From?

With the new research, the interest in Vitamin D is accelerating quickly. Low levels of Vitamin D can be the root cause of many problems. While it is impossible to get your Vitamin D levels from the sun all the time, we can get it through supplements or food.

Fish

If you love eating fish, you can opt for salmon as it contains good levels of Vitamin D. [145] If you consume 3.5 ounces of Salmon that is farmed, it will give 66% of the recommended dietary value of Vitamin D. Wild Salmon has even more levels of Vitamin D in them. However, the levels of Vitamin D can fluctuate with the time of the year.

Besides that, Herring is also considered a good source of Vitamin D. This is eaten globally and is often pickled or smoked. Though it is small in size, it is enriched with Vitamin D. Other than Herrings; Sardines also contains 24% of the required levels of Vitamin D. When you talk about Mackerel and Halibut; they also constitute Vitamin D. If you do not like the option of fresh fishes much, there is always canned tuna to save the day. Consisting of Vitamin D, canned tuna can help you get your Vitamin D levels.

Yolks

While fish is a good source of Vitamin D, there are other sources of it too. Eggs, for example, are nutritious food and contain Vitamin D. [146] The protein part is located in the egg whites,

---

[145] Leech, J. (2019). *11 Evidence-Based Health Benefits of Eating Fish.* Healthline. https://www.healthline.com/nutrition/11-health-benefits-of-fish

[146] Singh, S. (2022, June 15). *5 Nutritious Foods That Are Rich in Vitamin D.* TheQuint. https://www.thequint.com/fit/five-foods-rich-in-vitamin-d-eggs-mushrooms

while you can hunt for the fats, minerals, and vitamins in the yolk of the egg. If the chicken has an adequate amount of Vitamin D through the sunlight and the feed, it will result in the eggs having a higher claim of Vitamin D.

Mushrooms

Mushrooms are the only food that is rich in Vitamin D and is a non-animal food (of course, except for fortified food). Mushrooms can conduct the synthesis of Vitamin D when they are exposed to UV rays. While animals produce Vitamin D3, which is more effective than Vitamin D2, mushrooms tend to produce Vitamin D2. Wild mushrooms are a better source of Vitamin D2.

What are the Benefits of Vitamin D?

Vitamin D Helps In Weight Loss

People who have an increased weight possess a chance that they have a deficiency of Vitamin D. [147]A research was conducted where some people were given a diet plan to follow. Half of them were given supplements of Vitamin D, while others only had to follow the diet plan. It was seen that the people who consumed the supplements of Vitamin D lost more weight compared to those who did not consume the supplements of Vitamin D. You can consult your nutritionist or healthcare professional regarding it so that you can sort out the related problems to your weight.

Vitamin D Helps In Battling Depression

Vitamin D is considered essential in regulating mood; hence, it can help in managing depression too. People who were given Vitamin D supplements were seen to have an improvement in their mood. It also helps in soothing your anxiety and has a soothing effect on the body.

---

147 Low Vitamin D and Weight Gain: Is There a Connection? (2021, January 7). Healthline. https://www.healthline.com/nutrition/low-vitamin-d-and-weight-gain

It May Help In Battling Diseases
It helps in battling diseases. It aids in decreasing the risk of MS (Multiple Sclerosis).

Decreased levels of Vitamin D lead to a risk of heart disease, while adequate amounts of it can help deter the risk. [148]

Studies are going on for the effects of Vitamin D on flu and Covid-19. It is seen that sufficient levels of Vitamin D may help in keeping you safe from them.

It May Help In Supporting the Health of the Immune System
People with adequate amounts of Vitamin D are at a lesser risk of infections than people with a decreased rate of Vitamin D. Vitamin D also helps in battling autoimmune diseases that include Diabetes (type 1), inflammatory bowel disease, and rheumatoid arthritis. [149] Hence, sufficient consumption of this essential vitamin can be perfect for the health of your immune system.

---

[148] Kheiri, B., Abdalla, A., Osman, M., Ahmed, S., Hassan, M., & Bachuwa, G. (2018). Vitamin D deficiency and risk of cardiovascular diseases: a narrative review. *Clinical Hypertension, 24*. https://doi.org/10.1186/s40885-018-0094-4

[149] Ibid, 148

Importance of Vitamin E (Tocopherol)

What is Vitamin E?

This Vitamin is also known as Tocopherol. It is fat-soluble and exists in many forms. The form that is utilized by the body of humans is termed alpha-tocopherol. Vitamin holds immense importance because of its massive functions in the body. The main function of Vitamin E is to act as an antioxidant - due to this role, it hunts for the free radicals known as loose electrons. The reason that these free radicals are hunted is due to their damaging properties of it. The radicals tend to damage the body's cells, and Tocopherol prevents that from happening by hunting them down.

Other than that, one more important function conducted of Vitamin E is to improve the function of the immune system. Due to this, prevention is done against the clotting in the heart, and hence it can provide the risk of many diseases to some extent too.

These antioxidants were first introduced in the year 1980. This was when the scientists discovered that they could observe the participation of free radicals in the damage inflicted on the initial stages of artery-clogging atherosclerosis, which could also be a potential cause of cancer, loss of vision, and many other chronic diseases.

Vitamin E is an essential component that helps to battle against free radical damage. In a few conditions, Vitamin E is also known to decrease the production of free radicals in the body; but due to the contradicting studies, using high doses of Vitamin E to prevent chronic diseases is still not advised.

This Vitamin is also enriched with nutrients essential for our vision, skin health, brain, blood, and reproduction process.

When you consume Vitamin E solely for its antioxidant properties, you should know that the supplements of this Vitamin may not be as effective as the natural sources of Vitamin E in food. If the body does not have sufficient Vitamin E, it can even result in neuropathy (pain in the nerves of the body).

What Natural Sources Can You Get Vitamin E From?

Many foods are enriched with Vitamin E. Amongst them, there are olive oil, almonds, canola oil, and peanuts. You can also find Vitamin E in dairy, meat, margarine, fortified cereals, and leafy greens. [150]You can get oral supplements of Vitamin E in the form of drops or capsules. If you do not have adequate amounts of Vitamin E in your body, you can talk to your health care professional about Vitamin E supplements.

Beet Greens

While the beetroot is commonly eaten in most parts of the glove, the leaves or greens of the beetroot are not widely used. Most people might be surprised to know that the greens of beets are useful to consumers because they contain some levels of Vitamin E in them. You can use them in many forms, chop them up and use them in salads. You can also saute them in a little oil and enjoy.

Eating a hundred grams serving worth of beet greens will give you around 1.81 mg of Vitamin E. Beet greens not only contain Vitamin E but have more nutrients as well. These include Vitamin C and A, Fiber, Potassium, Calcium, and iron.

---

[150] Arnarson, A. (2017, May 24). *20 Foods That Are High in Vitamin E*. Healthline. https://www.healthline.com/nutrition/foods-high-in-vitamin-e

Trout

When it comes to fish, trout is an excellent source of Vitamin E. [151]If you ingest around 100 grams of trout, you will be able to attain around 2.15 mg worth of Vitamin E. Trout also consists of omega-3 fatty acids that are healthy. If you consume about a hundred grams of trout, it would contain around 21.1 grams of protein. Therefore, ensure to include this in your diet if you have a deficiency of Vitamin E. You can use it in many forms. Marinate it with the spices you love, fry them up, or bake them if you wish.

Spinach

Popeye has been known as a healthy food for a long time. It has many health benefits and also contains some levels of vitamin E in it. If you consume around a hundred grams of raw spinach, you can attain around 2.03 mg of Vitamin E through it. The same hundred grams of raw spinach will also contain Vitamin C, A, Potassium, and Fiber.

Avocados

Avocados are a healthy food that has a decreased amount of sugar. At the same time, they contain a lot of other nutrients in them. If you consume a hundred grams of avocado, you could get 2.07 mg of Vitamin E through it. Besides Vitamin E, the same hundred grams of avocado will also contain more nutrients like Vitamin C, potassium, etc. Due to this, they are considered to be healthy for humans. Avocados can be eaten in many forms; you can spread them on a toast or stuff them up; you can also season them up as per your liking and eat them. They can be consumed as a part of salads or can be ingested in the form of soups, too.

---

[151] *The 10 best foods high in vitamin E.* (2019, January 29). Www.medicalnewstoday.com.
https://www.medicalnewstoday.com/articles/324308#

Almonds

Almonds are one of the healthy nuts that can be consumed easily. They are very nutritious and beneficial for health.[152] When you consume around a hundred grams of almonds, you can obtain 25.63 mg of Vitamin E. You can eat almonds as a healthy snack, munch on roasted almonds, add them up when you are having your cereals, sprinkle them on the baked good, or opt for almond milk. Besides Vitamin E, almonds also contain proteins, magnesium, potassium, and fiber.

Peanuts

Peanuts are considered a popular snack and are eaten in many parts of the globe. If you consume a hundred grams of dry-roasted peanuts, you will get around 4.93 mg of Vitamin E through it.[153] The best thing to snack on is plain, dry-roasted peanuts, and if you like the ones with extra flavors and salt, you should rethink your decision. The plain dry-roasted ones are a healthier option than the salty ones. Along with 4.93 mg of Vitamin E, a hundred grams of peanuts also contain proteins, niacin, potassium, and fiber.

Oils

Some specific oils are enriched with Vitamin E.[154] While they contain Vitamin E, they do not contain many nutrients apart from calories and fat. Different oils have varying levels of Vitamin E in them.

1 tbsp of wheat germ Oil - 20.32 mg of Vitamin E

1 tbsp of Grapeseed Oil - 3.92 mg of Vitamin E

---

[152] Leech, J. (2018). *9 evidence-based health benefits of almonds*. Healthline. https://www.healthline.com/nutrition/9-proven-benefits-of-almonds
[153] *The 10 best foods high in vitamin E*. (2019, January 29). Www.medicalnewstoday.com. https://www.medicalnewstoday.com/articles/324308#peanuts
[154] Arnarson, A. (2017, May 24). *20 Foods That Are High in Vitamin E*. Healthline. https://www.healthline.com/nutrition/foods-high-in-vitamin-e

1 tbsp of Rice Bran Oil - 4.39 mg of Vitamin E

1 tbsp of Safflower Oil - 4.64 mg of Vitamin E

Hence, you can observe a good amount of Vitamin E in these four different oils.

What are the Benefits of Vitamin E?

Vitamin E has many benefits for the body. It is essential to the body, so it is important to ensure that your body has adequate levels of Vitamin E. Some benefits of Vitamin E are mentioned below:

Vitamin E Helps in Battling Oxidative Stress

There is a condition that occurs in the body due to the imbalance of the antioxidant defenses of the body, causing oxidative stress. [155] The production and storage of such compounds are termed ROS (Reactive Oxygen Species). The presence of these can lead to damage to the cells as well as increase the risk of disease in the body. Vitamin E is a robust antioxidant available in the body and helps battle this oxidative stress. According to some studies, it is also seen increased levels of Vitamin E have aided in decreasing the markers of this oxidative stress in the body. Furthermore, they have also helped boost the defense of some people's antioxidants.

Vitamin E Helps People with NAFLD

NAFLD stands for Non-Alcoholic Fatty Liver Disease. Fat may be accumulated in the liver of people who do not consume alcohol or consume a very small portion of it. Some research points to the findings that adequate vitamin E supplements may help improve people with NAFLD.

---

[155] Dix, M. (2017, December 13). *Everything You Should Know About Oxidative Stress*. Healthline; Healthline Media. https://www.healthline.com/health/oxidative-stress

Vitamin E Helps To Manage Dysmenorrhea
People who suffer from Dysmenorrhea are observed to have severe pain while menstruating. [156]It frequently occurs in the form of pelvic pain or cramps. Promising results have been projected due to the effects of Vitamin E on women, and the pain has been seen to be decreased before.

A study was conducted in 2021 that had women ingesting Vitamin E and Vitamin C for eight weeks. They were observed, and it was seen that the daily dosage of these vitamins had aided in decreasing the severity of the symptoms of Dysmenorrhea in women.

Vitamin E Help Decrease The Risk Of Heart Disease
This Vitamin has been seen to showcase promising results n decreasing the risk of heart disease in people. Hence taking Vitamin E supplements may reduce many heart problems.

---

[156] Cleveland Clinic. (2014). *What Is Dysmenorrhea / Menstrual Cramps | Cleveland Clinic: Health Library*. Cleveland Clinic. https://my.clevelandclinic.org/health/diseases/4148-dysmenorrhea

Importance of Vitamin K (Phylloquinone)

What is Vitamin K?

Vitamin K is also known as Phylloquinone. It is a vitamin that is fat-soluble in nature. It plays a role in the clotting of the blood, regulation of the calcium levels in the blood, and metabolism of the bones.[157]

Vitamin K is quite important as it helps in the production of prothrombin. For those of you who do not know what prothrombin is, it is a protein in the body and a clotting factor - and this helps in the metabolism of the bone. People who have been prescribed medication for blood thinning should not consume any additional dose of Vitamin K till they get advice from their healthcare professional. While the deficiency of this vitamin is rare, it is seen that its toxicity of it can lead to an extension in the time of clotting, and this can lead to excessive bleeding and even hemorrhage. There is another protein called Osteocalcin that is dependent on Vitamin K for the production of healthy tissues of the bones.

There are two types of Vitamin K. One is Vitamin K1, which comes from the plant. [158]This one is known as phylloquinone, also considered the main type of Vitamin K. This can be found in spinach, collard greens, kale, etc.

The second one is Vitamin K2, which is also termed menaquinone. Vitamin K2 or menaquinone can also be produced

---

[157] Calcitonin: What It Is, Function & Side Effects. (n.d.). Cleveland Clinic. https://my.clevelandclinic.org/health/articles/22330-calcitonin

[158] Pearson, K. (2017, September 15). *Vitamin K1 vs K2: What's the Difference?* Healthline; Healthline Media. https://www.healthline.com/nutrition/vitamin-k1-vs-k2

in the body by certain bacteria. This can occur in fermented foods as well as animal-based food.

Vitamin K can be found in many body parts, including the heart, brain, pancreas, bone, and liver. While it is fat-soluble in nature, it can be broken down in a quick manner and is excreted out of the body in the form of stool or urine. Due to this process, the toxicity of this vitamin is rare compared to other fat-soluble vitamins.

What Natural Sources Can You Get Vitamin K From?

Vitamin K can be found in many natural foods. Some of them are listed below.

Kale
If you consume half a cup of cooked kale, you will get 565 mcg of Vitamin K through it. Kale is an excellent source of Vitamin K. This also helps in allowing the proteins to go through the process of blood clotting. It is very important that your blood can clots because it protects your body from bleeding too much. Kale is considered to be a superfood as it is very nutritious. [159] Along with a good amount of Vitamin K, it is also enriched with folate, potassium, calcium, and other minerals and vitamins too. Kale is a healthy food that should be used in your diet so that you can get the nutrients out of it.

Soybeans
If you consume half a cup of roasted soybeans, it will contain around 43 mcg of Vitamins.

As we know, Vitamin K occurs in two forms - K1 and K2. K1 or phylloquinone is derived from plants, while K2 or menaquinone comes from fermented and animal-based foods. Soybeans have more of the K2 vitamins than the K1. [160]So you can incorporate soybeans into your diet to get an adequate amount of Vitamin K.

Sauerkraut

Half a cup of sauerkraut will give you around 56 mcg of Vitamin K. You can stack up sauerkraut in your hot dogs and at it. Along with Vitamin K, you will get your proteins as well. You can find them in many local eateries.

Asparagus

Half a cup of asparagus has 72 mcg of Vitamin K. You can pair it up with a little bit of olive oil, the ad you can get half of your required consumption of vitamin K. You can not pack up a lot of vitamin K-rich food in one day as it will not do any good. The body flushes out the vitamin K from your body even though it is a fat-soluble vitamin. [161]So, you can intake it on a daily basis and consume food that contains Vitamin K in it. Asparagus is a good source of Vitamin K and can be included in the diet to keep up the levels of Vitamin K.

Lettuce

Consuming half a head of iceberg or one cup of romaine will give you 60 mcg of Vitamin K. Lettuce is commonly used as a popular dietary intake in many parts of the world. It is a part of many salads and is found easily in many grocery stores as well. It includes varieties like romaine, bibb, green leaf, and of course, iceberg. So, you can use up the lettuce in your regular diet in various forms, and this will help in keeping good levels of Vitamin K in your body.

Broccoli

Half a cup of cooked broccoli will lead to 85 mcg of Vitamin K. You can prepare broccoli using various methods. You can add a little bit of canola oil or olive oil, as it can help in boosting the

---

[160] Pearson, K. (2017, September 15). Vitamin K1 vs K2: What's the Difference? Healthline; Healthline Media.
https://www.healthline.com/nutrition/vitamin-k1-vs-k2

vitamin K levels in your body. A tablespoon of canola or olive oil is calculated to contain ten mcg of Vitamin K.

Brussels sprouts

Half a cup of cooked Brussels sprouts pack around 150 mcg of Vitamin K. While cooking Brussels sprouts with kids in the house may arouse some protests from the little ones; some recipes can really give a twist to them. You can try adding Sriracha aioli and garlic and making crispy Brussel Sprouts.

Turnip greens

Half a cup of cooked turnip greens can give around 425 mcg of Vitamin K. In the southeastern parts of the United States; these Turnip greens are cooked as quite a popular side dish. They are rich in calcium, and due to this, it also helps in strengthening the bones. [162]Apart from that, beet greens and mustard greens also contain Vitamin K. The turnip has a bulbous part that grows underground, which is nutritious as well.

Collard greens

You can get vitamin K-rich food in your diet to keep yourself safe from this problem. Ingesting half a cup of collard greens can help get 530 mcg of Vitamin K. Along with clotting, and this vitamin also helps in the growth of bone. Some studies have been conducted that show that the reduced level of Vitamin K is linked with the initiation of osteoporosis.

Pumpkin

Consuming half a cup of canned pumpkin leads to 20 mcg of Vitamin K. Have it in your diet and get an adequate amount of Vitamin K through it. Pumpkin in your diet can help maintain the levels of Vitamin K in the body. [163]This can be beneficial for the body as it helps in clotting the blood as well as aids in the metabolism of bone.

---

[162] *Turnips: Health benefits, nutrition, and dietary tips*. (2019, November 4). Www.medicalnewstoday.com.
https://www.medicalnewstoday.com/articles/284815

[163] *Pumpkin: Nutrition, Benefits, and How to Eat It*. (2021, August 26). Healthline. https://www.healthline.com/nutrition/pumpkin-nutrition-review#

Pickles

While the body can make Vitamin K2 on its own, we need to keep it in our diet. If you consume one cucumber dill, you get 25 mcg of Vitamin K. So, people who love eating pickles can benefit from it. The best thing is that the pickles have very low calories, which helps make them healthy and crunchy. [164]

Edamame

Eating around half a cup of boiled edamame will give you around 25 mcg of Vitamin K. Japanese use it as a part of their cuisines. When we talk about edamame, they are basically soybeans that occur in pods. They can be used as a quick, crunchy, and delicious snack by adding some light pepper and salt to them.

Blueberries

If you love blueberries, you would be glad to know that they also contain a certain level of Vitamin K. If you eat around half a cup of blueberries, you will get 14 mcg of Vitamin K. While all the others have been vegetables yet, this is one fruit that contains some Vitamin K in it

Pine nuts

Consuming one ounce of pine nuts will give you 15 mcg of Vitamin K. You can use them in various ways. You can toss them up in a salad and add a crunchy twist to it. You can also eat cashews as they also contain Vitamin K.

Eating up an ounce of dry-roasted cashews will provide around ten mcg of Vitamin K.

What are the Benefits of Vitamin K?

Vitamin K Helps in the Healing Of The Wounds

While blood clots may seem bad at times, they are not all bad. When you are hurt and get a cut or a scrape, there are specific proteins in the blood that cause the clotting of the blood would

---

[164] Leech, J. (2018, September 21). *Vitamin K2: Everything You Need to Know.* Healthline; Healthline Media. https://www.healthline.com/nutrition/vitamin-k2

stop the bleeding. [165]These proteins are reliant on Vitamin K for the clotting process.

Due to this, Vitamin K helps alter the blood's liquidy properties to a gel-like and sticky texture so that it can harden up to form a scab. If this process did not take place, an injury to the skin could cause you to bleed very much, probably to death. People suffering from or who take blood thinners may also experience major difficulty in clotting their blood. You can talk to your healthcare professional and ask about Vitamin K in your diet. If you need to maintain your diet of Vitamin K, they can guide you in regards to that.

Vitamin K Helps in The Prevention of Osteoporosis
While the link with osteoporosis has always been inclined towards vitamin D and calcium levels, Vitamin K also plays an important part in preventing osteoporosis. There are specified proteins that depend on Vitamin K for the proper health of the bones. There is a process known as carboxylation that is supposed to occur for the growth of bone. Here, the Vitamin K vitamin is supposed to be present for an enzyme named gamma-glutamyl carboxylase. The presence of the vitamin helps in the working of osteocalcin, which aids in the process of the growth of bone.

While it has an essential role in the metabolism of bone, there is not enough evidence to claim that Vitamin K decreases the risk of bone fractures. While studies also claim that a sufficient amount of Vitamin K can help in the prevention of bone loss as well as reduce the fractures in the hips of elderly women and men.

Osteoporosis can cause many hindrances in performance and daily chores. So, in order to prevent it, Vitamin K is thought to be a good addition.

---

[165] *The Blood Clotting Process: What Happens if You Have a Bleeding Disorder.* (2020). HemAware. https://hemaware.org/bleeding-disorders-z/blood-clotting-process-what-happens-if-you-have-bleeding-disorder

Vitamin K Decreases the Risks of Heart Disease

The calcification in your blood vessels and the risk of a cardiovascular event are very closely linked. [166]In a study, it was observed that there was a 400 percent increase in the risk of cardiovascular diseases in the case of calcification in any arterial wall. Contrary to this, sufficient levels of vitamin K have been linked with a reduced risk of heart disease in humans.

Vitamin K Helps In Reducing The Blood Pressure

You may want to keep your vitamin K levels sorted as it helps keep you safe from very high blood pressure. If [167]the blood pressure is adequate, it can also help lower the risk of cardiovascular diseases. Hypertension has been linked with low levels of Vitamin K, and Vitamin D. An increase in both systolic and diastolic pressures has been observed due to insufficient levels of Vitamin D and Vitamin K.

Vitamin K helps in the regulation of minerals in your blood. Due to vascular calcification, the calcium and other minerals in the blood tend to block the flow of blood with age. When we get sufficient levels of vitamin K, it helps block the minerals due to mineralization and helps reduce blood pressure.

Vitamin K Helps in the Improvement of the Memory of Older Adults

According to studies, it is seen that increased levels of Vitamin K, particularly Vitamin K1 or Phylloquinone, help in the improvement of verbal episodic memory. [168]That is one more benefit that can be quite important in the improvement of memory in people, especially the older ages. Hence, adequate levels of Vitamin K are required for this. At older ages, people can suffer

---

[166] Wu, M., Rementer, C., & Giachelli, C. M. (2013). Vascular Calcification: an Update on Mechanisms and Challenges in Treatment. *Calcified Tissue International, 93*(4), 365–373. https://doi.org/10.1007/s00223-013-9712-z

[167] Ware, M. (2018, January 22). *Vitamin K: Health benefits, daily intake, and sources.* Www.medicalnewstoday.com. https://www.medicalnewstoday.com/articles/219867

[168] Alisi, L., Cao, R., De Angelis, C., Cafolla, A., Caramia, F., Cartocci, G., Librando, A., & Fiorelli, M. (2019). The Relationships Between Vitamin K and Cognition: A Review of Current Evidence. *Frontiers in Neurology, 10.* https://doi.org/10.3389/fneur.2019.00239

from memory problems, so they can remember things easily, Vitamin K can help improve it. It can help make your memory better.

These are all the benefits of Vitamin K on the body. Some of them are still under observation and are being researched thoroughly to get the results. If you want to reap the benefits of Vitamin K, you should have a sufficient amount of it in the body. Due to this, your body can perform all the functions better so that you do not have to suffer through the troubles that can happen due to the deficiency of Vitamin K.

How Do Vitamins Work?

There are two main types of vitamins on the basis of their solubility. One is the water-soluble vitamins, while the other ones are known as the fat-soluble ones. Hence, the working of both kinds of vitamins varies a bit. Here, we are going to discover how vitamins work.

The Working of Water-Soluble Vitamins

The water-soluble vitamins are known to be stacked in portions of food that are watery in nature. When you consume it, you are able to get the water-soluble vitamins in your bloodstream. As your food goes through the process of breaking down during the digestive phase, these water-soluble vitamins get directly dissolved into the bloodstream.[169] The supplement dissolves in the same way in the body as well.

Since your body consists mostly of water, most water-soluble vitamins can easily transport into the body without much problem.

Your kidneys are responsible for regulating the proper levels of water-soluble vitamins in the body. The kidney ensures that the excess level of water-soluble vitamins is excreted out of the body through the urine. All the different vitamins have their own functions that they perform; amongst them, one of the most important functions is to help in freeing the energy that is found in the food that you consume. Other than that, it also helps maintain the health of the tissues.

---

[169] Helpguide. (2019, June 26). *HelpGuide.org*. HelpGuide.org. https://www.helpguide.org/harvard/vitamins-and-minerals.htm

The Working Of Fat-Soluble Vitamins

These are not excreted through the urine; rather, they are stored. Mostly, you can find them stored in the adipose tissues of the body.[170] As they are fat-soluble in nature, they do not get absorbed into the bloodstream. Instead of the bloodstream, they are absorbed into the small intestines through the lacteals. This process is done with the help of chylomicrons that transport them throughout the lymphatic system and then set to release them into the bloodstream.

---

[170] *Fat-Soluble Vitamins the Good and the Bad What are Fat-Soluble Vitamins?* (n.d.).
https://depts.washington.edu/ceeh/downloads/Fast%20Facts%20Fat%20Soluble%20Vitamins%20063015.pdf

Importance of Vitamins

If you want to ensure a healthy lifestyle, you would have to make sure that you listen to the requirements of your body. In order to stay active and nourished, you will need to choose the correct nutrients for your body. The vitamins in your diet can help you get a step closer to achieving your goals of a healthy body.

Vitamins are considered important nutrients due to their expansive range of roles in the body. Due to this, you need to make sure that you are getting a sufficient amount of these vitamins. There is a need to balance the intake of these vitamins - you can not have too few of them or too much of them; both conditions can harm your body in one way or the other.

The best way to get adequate vitamins in your body is by eating a well-balanced and healthy diet. If the vitamin levels remain low after that, you can always ask your healthcare professional about the usage of vitamin supplements in your daily routine.

Vitamins Are Essential For the Human Body

The human body produces muscle, skin, and bone on a regular basis. The flow of blood in the body aids in carrying oxygen along with nutrients from one place to another. [171]This blood also sends out signals that radiate through the pathways of the brain and the body. With that, instructions are also sent in the form of chemical messengers; this is done to help in maintaining your life.

To carry out these functions properly, the human body needs specific raw materials, such as minerals, vitamins, and dietary components. The body requires these but can not produce them on its own, so they should be utilized in our diet.

---

[171]Better Health Channel. (2012, September 30). *Circulatory system*. Vic.gov.au.
https://www.betterhealth.vic.gov.au/health/conditionsandtreatments/circulatory-system

The vitamins combined with minerals are able to perform many roles in the body. They help in healing wounds, strengthening the bones, and giving a boost to your immune system. Also, food is converted into energy due to their help, and the damage in the cells is also repaired. Hence, they serve as very vital nutrition for our body.

When you are trying to learn about vitamins, there may be a time when your mind is spinning with the alphabet soup that has been created due to them. While they can be quite confusing, they are not that hard to understand. Do not worry about the spinning letters; you will get the hang of it.

Previously, we have described all the vitamins in detail so that you get a complete understanding of the importance of each and every vitamin in the human body.

Why Are These Micronutrients Important?

Vitamins are known as micronutrients as they are needed in minute amounts by the body. [172]If those minor requirements are not met, it can result in a few diseases that can occur due to the deficiencies of vitamins.

Blindness

In some countries that are still in the phase of development, people have been seen losing sight and becoming blind due to the deficiency of Vitamin A. So, blindness is one of the problems that can occur due to insufficient levels of Vitamin A.

Scurvy

If you do not get sufficient doses of Vitamin C, this could result in bleeding of the gums and also scurvy[173]. So, make sure that you keep your levels of vitamins in check.

---

[172] Harvard. (2019, February 15). *Vitamins*. The Nutrition Source. https://www.hsph.harvard.edu/nutritionsource/vitamins

[173] Crosta, P. (2017, December 5). Scurvy: Symptoms, causes, treatment, andprevention.Www.medicalnewstoday.com.
https://www.medicalnewstoday.com/articles/155758

Rickets

If you do not have adequate levels of Vitamin D in the body, this can result in rickets, which causes your bones to become soft, porous, and fragile. This could be a leading cause of deformities in the skeletal structure of the human body. Due to these reasons, In the United States of America, milk has been fortified with Vitamin D for a long time.

So, if you do not have proper levels of these micronutrients in the body, it can be quite problematic and harmful.

On the other hand, sufficient levels of these micronutrients can be very beneficial for the human body. If your body has a significant amount of these vitamins, you can get many benefits.

Prevention of Birth Defects

Ask your healthcare professional if you need folic acid supplements during your pregnancy. These can help in the prevention of spinal and brain defects in the fetus. Hence, it is termed as very important.

Strengthened Bones

You require Vitamin D and Vitamin K in adequate measurements in your body; this is because your body needs them to keep your bones strong, which will help in protecting them against fractures. [174]

Maintaining The Health Of Your Teeth

They also maintain the health of your teeth. This is why they are considered to be quite important too.

---

[174] Sunyecz, J. A. (2008). The use of calcium and vitamin D in the management of osteoporosis. *Therapeutics and Clinical Risk Management*, 4(4), 827–836. https://doi.org/10.2147/tcrm.s3552

What is the need for Vitamin Supplements?

When you inspect the market, you will see around ninety thousand different types of supplements. That is a huge number that is placed on the racks. Many vitamin supplements are curated in the laboratory.[175] On the contrary, some of them are also emanated from natural sources. One of the most common natural sources is fish oil.

Not all people need to take supplements for vitamins. Some can get their vitamins from their diet; this can only happen if you eat a well-balanced diet. The vitamins are essential for the body and aid the body in working perfectly. Many people have opted for an intake of supplements on a regular basis.

You need to know that just as low levels of vitamins can be dangerous, so can their excessive levels. So, make sure you consult your health care professional for the recommended dose and the time span you should take them.

Do You Need To Take Supplements Of Vitamins?

Whether or not you should start taking Vitamin supplements depends on your healthcare professional analysis and recommendation. It will help if you consult your healthcare professional about this. They will guide you as per the levels of Vitamins in your body. Since the vitamins can also be taken through your diet, it is considered a more appropriate means of getting your vitamin levels sorted.

Supplements of vitamins have been linked with an improvement in thinking, betterment in the health of the heart, and a strengthened immune system. They help take over the

---

[175] *How vitamin is made - ingredients of, making, history, used, processing, components, steps, product.* (2014). Madehow.com. http://www.madehow.com/Volume-3/Vitamin.html

deficiencies of the vitamin level in your body. Although, many benefits have not been scientifically proven yet.

Supplements of Vitamin D

In the months starting from March and extending towards September, people can get the doses of Vitamin D through the sunlight they receive. It can also be balanced through a good diet. The sun lacks sufficient amounts of vitamin D in autumn and winter. However, getting an adequate amount of Vitamin D from the diet is not an easy task. Hence, supplements can be used then. Mostly, ten micrograms of Vitamin D supplements are perfect for regular use but still contact your health care professional for this. Normally, even breastfeeding or pregnant women can also have these supplements.

Some people are more prone to suffer from a deficiency of Vitamin D. They might have to take supplements for it around the year.

Folic Acid And Pregnancy

When women are pregnant or trying to conceive, folic acid is often recommended for them. [176]It is best to consult a healthcare professional for this, but four hundred micrograms of this supplement are generally considered safe for both - the mother and the fetus. This can be taken for a period of twelve weeks when pregnant. The supplements of folic acid should be introduced into your diet even before you are pregnant. Hence you can start taking them when you stop using contraceptives. Due to folic acid, neural birth defects like spina bifida can be prevented in babies. [177]

Vitamin A, C, and D Supplements

It is considered safe to have supplements for vitamins A, C, and D, but you should not do this without consulting your

---

[176] *Folic Acid and Pregnancy (for Parents) - Nemours KidsHealth.* (n.d.). Kidshealth.org. https://kidshealth.org/en/parents/preg-folic-acid.html

[177] CDC. (2020, January 2). *Folic Acid Helps Prevent Some Birth Defects.* Centers for Disease Control and Prevention. https://www.cdc.gov/ncbddd/folicacid/features/folic-acid-helps-prevent-some-birth-defects.html

healthcare professional first. The supplements for vitamins are even considered safe for children and can be given to them to battle several health conditions.

Are The Supplements of Vitamins A Safe Option?

When you are using them in moderation, most supplements are considered to be safe. The toxicity of anything can be hazardous to health, and it is the same with these supplements. You need to consult a healthcare advisor and ask them about the recommended dose on a regular basis. Also, you should know the time duration for which you should be using them. It is quite possible to get an adverse reaction from the supplements if taken at the wrong time. There are around 23,000 cases of emergency every year in the hospital, which are linked to the use of nutritional supplements. So, to avoid them, make sure you have a consultation session beforehand.

Always let your physician know all your history and provide them with the details about the supplements. Also, make sure you discard the old vitamins that are not used.

The FDA (Food and Drug Administration) is responsible for ensuring the safety of supplements for use. [178] While the prescribed drugs go through vigilant testing processes, supplements do not go through such sharp measures.

What is Better - Supplements or a Balanced Diet?

The body is more apt to absorb the nutrients from the diet as compared to supplements.[179] So, a balanced diet is a better solution to keep your vitamin levels balanced. You can have vegetables, fruits, cheese, whole grains, poultry, fish, and even lean meats - these help in stacking up your vitamins in the body.

---

[178] https://www.fda.gov/food/information-consumers-using-dietary-supplements/questions-and-answers-dietary-supplements

[179] *Vitamin D foods: Fruits, vegetables, and other sources.* (2019, February 28). Www.medicalnewstoday.com. https://www.medicalnewstoday.com/articles/324590#summary

Due to these foods, the absorption capability is accelerated, allowing your body to use the ratio of vitamins it has efficiently.

Hence, a healthy diet is much better than using supplements.

Do Vegetarians Require Supplements?

Vegetables contain many vitamins, and due to that, you would not need supplements. Your body would be getting adequate nutrients through the diet that you are getting. If you think you should opt for vitamin supplements, you can always talk to your healthcare advisor before attempting something.

Do Vegans Require Supplements?

People who are vegan are most likely to have a deficiency of Vitamin B12. To address this issue, many foods consumed, especially by vegans, are fortified with Vitamin B12. [180]One example of it is almond milk. This milk is fortified with Vitamin B12 to help ensure that your levels of this vitamin remain sufficient. Even with this, there might be a requirement for a supplement sometimes. Your healthcare professional can guide you better regarding it. Talk to them and let them know everything so they can guide you accordingly.

---

[180] *Vitamin B-12 foods for vegetarians and vegans.* (2018, January 7). Www.medicalnewstoday.com.
https://www.medicalnewstoday.com/articles/320524#foods-for-vegans

The Optimum Daily Intake of Vitamins

There is a specific amount of vitamins that Human beings need for their body. If you get more than that, they can suffer from its toxicity, which can be dangerous. If they do not get sufficient amounts of vitamins in their body, it can also be a risky thing for the body. Hence, you must ensure that your body has the required amounts of vitamins.

RDA - This is a term you will use when talking about the needed doses of vitamins. It stands for Recommended Dietary Allowance. [181] AI is another term that is commonly used. This means Adequate Intake of the vitamins that help keep you healthy and nutritious. These have been customized according to the need of men and women and are also distinguished on the basis of ages.

The UL determines the maximized amount of vitamins that you can have without the risk of an overdose. UL stands for Tolerable Upper Intake Level. If you go beyond the capacity of UL, you can suffer from many problems, side effects, or even the possibility of an overdose.

The FDA, known as the Food and Drug Administration, also uses a specific means of measurement. This is termed DV. DV stands for the Daily Value. You may be able to find the DV on the labels of foods as well as supplements.

The RDA (Recommended Dietary Allowance) and DV (Daily Value) are set so that you can easily prevent disease due to toxicity or lack of nutrition.[182] Here, we will see the number of vitamins needed by the body to stay healthy.

---

[181] Allowances, N. R. C. (US) S. on the T. E. of the R. D. (1989). Definition and Applications. In *www.ncbi.nlm.nih.gov*. National Academies Press (US). https://www.ncbi.nlm.nih.gov/books/NBK234926/

[182] Allowances, N. R. C. (US) S. on the T. E. of the R. D. (1989). Definition and Applications. In *www.ncbi.nlm.nih.gov*. National Academies Press (US). https://www.ncbi.nlm.nih.gov/books/NBK234926/

Vitamin A - Retinol

These include retinoids and carotenoids like retinyl steers, retinoic acid, retinal, and of course, retinol. Some are even known as preformed vitamin A. They are quite important for vision. They also help in decreasing the risk of prostate cancer. They aid in keeping the skin and tissues healthy and play a significant role in the growth of bone. It also helps in giving a boost to the immune system.

In males, the Recommended Daily Allowance for each day is **900 mcg**. For women, the RDA stands at **700 mcg.** The UL or Upper Limit stands at **3000 micrograms**. There are many natural sources of vitamin A, like beef liver, shrimp, eggs, fish, butter, milk, etc.

Vitamin B1 - Thiamin

This vitamin helps convert food into energy that can be used by the body. Other than that, it is also important for your muscles, brain, skin, and hair health. Also, nerve function is affected by it, so we need to ensure a sufficient amount of this vitamin.

The males require a Recommended Dietary Allowance of 1.2 mg of Vitamin B1 while women can 1.1 mg of it. [183]The UL is not really known of this as of yet. You can get this vitamin from natural food sources like brown rice, pork chops, ham, soymilk, etc. Nutritious foods mostly have some levels of Vitamin B1 in them.

Vitamin B2 - Riboflavin

The body requires it in order to keep the skin healthy. It is also needed for keeping up blood, hair, and brain health. This vitamin also helps in the conversion of food into energy.

The Required Dietary Allowance for each day for males is 1.3 mg. For females, the RDA is 1.1 mg. the Upper Limit is still not known for riboflavin. You can get Vitamin B2 from many natural

---

[183] Harvard T.H. Chan. (2019, July 8). *Thiamin – Vitamin B1*. The Nutrition Source. https://www.hsph.harvard.edu/nutritionsource/vitamin-b1/

sources like eggs, milk, cheese, yogurt, vegetables, fortified cereals, and whole grains.[184] In America, most people have sufficient levels of this particular vitamin.

Vitamin B3 - Niacin

Vitamin B1 is also known as niacin. It helps in the conversion of food into energy. It is considered important for the health of the blood cells, nervous system, and brain.

The Recommended Dietary Allowance for males per day is 16 mg. For women, it is a bit reduced and falls at 16 mg. The UL level of niacin (Vitamin B3) is 35 mg.

Some natural sources of Vitamin B3 are poultry, meat, fish, whole grains, mushrooms, peanuts, potatoes, butter, etc. Your body also makes some niacin with the help of the amino acid tryptophan; this process is done with the help of Vitamin B6.

Vitamin B5 - Pantothenic Acid

Vitamin B5 is also known as pantothenic acid and helps convert food into a form of energy for the body. [185]It helps make lipids, a steroid hormone, hemoglobin, and neurotransmitters.

The males and females both have a Required Dietary Allowance (RDA) of 5 mg per day. The UL level is not known for now.

Natural foods also have Vitamin B5 in them. Some examples are eggs, chicken, whole grains, mushrooms, tomato, broccoli, etc. If a deficiency of Vitamin B5 occurs, you can also experience burning in the feet and other neurologic symptoms.

---

[184] *Riboflavin – Vitamin B2.* (2020, July 24). The Nutrition Source. https://www.hsph.harvard.edu/nutritionsource/riboflavin-vitamin-b2/

[185] *Vitamin B5 (Pantothenic acid) Information | Mount Sinai - New York.* (n.d.). Mount Sinai Health System. https://www.mountsinai.org/health-library/supplement/vitamin-b5-pantothenic-acid

Vitamin B6 - Pyridoxine

Vitamin B6 is also known as pyridoxine. It helps in reducing the levels of homocysteine in the body.[186] This can help battle the occurrence of heart disease. It also helps in the conversion of the amino acid tryptophan to niacin and also, serotonin. Due to this, you can observe a betterment in your sleep patterns, mood, and as well as your appetite.

In males of 30 years to 50 years, the required dietary allowance for a day is 1.3 mg. In women, the RDA is 1.5 mg.

Some natural sources of Vitamin b6 are poultry, legumes, fish, meat, tofu, etc. This vitamin is deficient in many people.

Vitamin B12 - Cobalamin

Vitamin B12 is also known as cobalamin. It lowers the levels of homocysteine in the body and also helps in the development of new cells. Other than that, this vitamin is known to break down some of the amino acids and fatty acids too. Vitamin B12 also helps in the protection of the cells of the nerves and ensures their healthy development of them. Furthermore, it also helps in making DNA and red blood cells.

The men and women both require a Required Dietary Allowance of 2.4 mcg per day.

You can find this vitamin in many natural sources like fish, cheese, meat, eggs, fortified cereal, etc.[187] As people grow older, they may lose the capability to absorb Vitamin B12 efficiently.

---

[186] Streit, L. (2018, October). *9 Health Benefits of Vitamin B6 (Pyridoxine)*. Healthline; Healthline Media. https://www.healthline.com/nutrition/vitamin-b6-benefits

[187] Semeco, A. (2018, May 3). *Top 12 Foods That Are High in Vitamin B12*. Healthline; Healthline Media. https://www.healthline.com/nutrition/vitamin-b12-foods

Vitamin B7 - Biotin

Vitamin B7 is also known as biotin. This vitamin is proficient at the synthesis of glucose and helps in the breaking down of a couple of fatty acids too. It helps in the conversion of food into energy as well.

The men and women both have a Required Dietary Allowance of 30 mcg per day. Many natural foods have biotin in them, like eggs, meat, whole grains, etc. it is even made in the gastrointestinal tract with the help of bacteria.

Vitamin C - Ascorbic Acid

Vitamin C is also called ascorbic acid. It aids in the reduction of the risk of many cancers, which include the esophagus, stomach, breast, and mouth. It may also help in the protection against cataracts.

Men have a Recommended Dietary Allowance of 90 mg; for women, it is 75 mg daily. It is found in natural sources like fruits, strawberries, broccoli, bell peppers, etc.

Vitamin D - Calciferol

Vitamin D is commonly known as calciferol. It is very important as it helps maintain the blood levels of phosphorus and calcium in the body. The maintained levels help make the bones strong in the human body. Vitamin D also helps in the formation of bones and teeth. Hence it is a vital vitamin that is needed by the body. Getting enough vitamin D can help decrease non-spinal fractures.

The Required Dietary Allowance for Vitamin D with respect to each day is 15 mcg. This is for people who are in the age group of 31 to 70 years. For men and women exceeding the age of 71, 20 mcg of Vitamin D is required by the body to carry out the functions properly. The Upper Limit of Vitamin D is 50 mcg, which should not be exceeded.

Some natural sources of Vitamin D are fortified milk, margarine, fatty fish, fortified cereals, etc. The human body uses

Vitamin D to make sunlight, but living in northern climates, you may not get sufficient time in the sun - this can lead to a deficiency of Vitamin D.

Vitamin E - Alpha Tocopherol

It is also known as alpha-tocopherol. This vitamin behaves as an antioxidant and helps neutralize unstable molecules. It also helps in the protection of Vitamin A from undergoing damage. The UL of Vitamin E is 1000 mg. The men and women both require an RDA of 15 mg.

It is found in many natural sources like salad dressing, margarine, vegetables, leafy greens, and whole grains. [188]

Vitamin B9 - Folic Acid, Folate

Vitamin B9 is also known as folate or folic acid. Women are recommended folic acid in their pregnancy as it helps prevent spine and brain defects that can occur at birth. It is important for cell development. This vitamin also helps in the reduction of homocysteine levels which helps in preventing the disease of the heart. Also, a sufficient amount of it can help reduce the risk of colon cancer. It also helps in reducing the risk of breast cancer in women.

The Required Dietary Allowance of Vitamin B9 is 400 mcg in both men and women. [189]The UL of it is 1000 mcg. There are many natural sources of this vitamin; these include fortified cereals, fortified grains, okra, broccoli, legumes, turnip, spinach, asparagus, chickpeas, orange juice, etc. Many people do not get a proper amount of this vitamin.

---

[188] Arnarson, A. (2017, May 24). *20 Foods That Are High in Vitamin E*. Healthline. https://www.healthline.com/nutrition/foods-high-in-vitamin-e

[189]Harvard School of Public Health. (2012, September 18). *Folate (Folic Acid) – Vitamin B9*. The Nutrition Source. https://www.hsph.harvard.edu/nutritionsource/folic-acid/

Vitamin K - Phylloquinone

Vitamin K is also called phylloquinone. It helps in the clotting of the blood by activating calcium and proteins. It also helps in preventing the risk of fractures in the hips. The males have a Required Dietary allowance of 120 mcg per day, while women have an RDA of 90 mcg for one day.

The UL of Vitamin K is still not known. Some natural sources of Vitamin K are liars, eggs, broccoli, kale, sprouts, etc. A bacteria in your intestine helps make a form of Vitamin K in your body; This fulfills half of the requirements of your body.

What Are Minerals?

Minerals are those inorganic solids that occur naturally and have a definite chemical composition.[190] Along with it, they also possess a regular structure of atoms. This is the most basic point that gives rise to all their other properties.

We are going to be learning about some physical properties of minerals.

Hardness - This makes them resistant to scratches.

Tenacity - This provides resistance to any impact.

Cleavage - The ability of some crystals to split at the point of weak bonding of atoms

Specific gravity - The relative density of it

Lustre - The Effect Of Minerals On Light

Refractive Index

Minerals occur in many different shapes and sizes. You can see some huge crystals, like quartz, that come from Brazilian pegmatites. Some are so tiny that the human eye can not see them. One of the small minerals is Chalcedony, also known as a microcrystalline.

The minerals are of many different colors. They can be made up of one single element or be an amalgamation of more elements - known as chemical compounds. Carbon, silver, and gold possess the ability to form elements on their own. This is why they are termed native elements. One mineral is your ordinary kitchen salt which is formed by the presence of chlorine and sodium ions.

---

[190] https://nbmg.unr.edu/_docs/ScienceEducation/Activities/WhatIsAMineral.pdf

The ions, molecules, and atoms that create a mineral are in well-defined geometrical shapes called crystal lattices. The shape of the crystal is present due to the structure of the crystal lattice.

How the atoms merge determines if the minerals would exfoliate or laminate. The hardness of the crystals is determined according to the Mohs scale. You can see soft minerals at the beginning that can be easily scratched with the help of a nail; these include calcite, chalk, and talc. At the end of the scale, you will notice hard minerals like diamonds. The diamond is known as the hardest mineral on the earth.

Why Are Minerals Important?

In order to stay healthy, you need to have minerals in your life. There are many different things that minerals do for the body. These include the proper working of your body's heart, muscles, and bones. Other than these, minerals are also important for creating hormones and enzymes in the human body.

When we talk about minerals, you can find two types of them. One type of mineral is known as trace minerals, while the others are called macrominerals.[191] You need to consume a larger amount of macrominerals to fulfill the requirements of the body, while you need a smaller amount of trace minerals in your body. The macrominerals include sodium, potassium, calcium, magnesium, phosphorus, chloride, and sulfur. Trace minerals include manganese, iodine, iron, copper, selenium, fluoride, cobalt, and zinc.[192]

You can get adequate minerals in your body by eating a well-balanced diet enriched with these minerals. There are some cases where the doctor may also recommend a supplement for the minerals. People who are going through some health problem or are taking specific medication may be required to take less intake of minerals too. For instance, people suffering from chronic kidney disease are recommended to limit the food with a high amount of potassium in it.

---

[191] News-Medical. (2019, February 27). *Macrominerals and Trace Minerals in the Diet*. News-Medical.net.
https://www.newsmedical.net/health/Macrominerals-and-Trace-Minerals-in-the-Diet.aspx

[192] Ibid.

Essential Minerals That Your Body Needs

Your body needs some minerals so that it can carry out all its functions in a proper manner. If there are insufficient levels of some minerals in the body, it may lead to a critical health condition. So, make sure that you take proper intake of minerals for your body. Some essential minerals that are needed by the body are mentioned below.

Calcium

Calcium is an essential mineral for the human body. This is due to the fact that calcium helps in building bones and teeth and also keeps them strong. Calcium is also vital for the contraction of muscles, clotting of the blood, transmission in the nerve cells, signaling of the cells, and regulating the metabolism in the body. [193]

If there is an insufficient amount of calcium in the body, this can lead to fragile bones and increase the risk of fracture. There are many natural sources of calcium, like dairy products, milk, dates, greens, broccoli, cashew, and parsley.

Sodium

Sodium is also an essential mineral that is required by the human body. It helps in the contraction of the muscle and helps in controlling the balance of fluid in the body.[194] Other than that, sodium helps in the conduction of nerve impulses in the body, and hence it is quite an important mineral. The most common dietary

---

[193] US), M., A Catharine Ross, Taylor, C. L., Yaktine, A. L., & B, H. (2011). *Overview of Calcium*. Nih.gov; National Academies Press (US). https://www.ncbi.nlm.nih.gov/books/NBK56060/

[194] West, H. (2018, October 24). *Electrolytes: Definition, Functions, Imbalance and Sources*. Healthline. https://www.healthline.com/nutrition/electrolytes

source of sodium is table salt. It should be kept in mind that we should be taking the salt in moderation and prevent the excessive use of it.

Potassium

Potassium is needed in adequate amounts by the body as it also plays a vital role in the body. It helps maintain the fluid balance in the body and helps deal with nerve impulse conduction and the contraction of the muscles. Potassium is known to support the health of the brain and also minimizes the risk of a stroke. If a person has low levels of potassium in their body, they can experience problems like brain damage, edema, and irregular heartbeats.

You can get potassium from natural food sources like bananas, avocados, sweet potatoes, dates, and beets.

Chloride

The chloride in the human body works alongside sodium in order to maintain fluid balance. [195]It also helps in the formation of HCL - hydrochloric acid in the stomach - which is used to help with digestion and helps in sustaining the electrical neutrality of the human body.

Regarding the diet, you can find chloride in table salt, celery, tomatoes, and lettuce.

Magnesium

This mineral is crucial as it behaves as a cofactor in many reactions that are enzymatic in nature. Other than that, magnesium is also required for the synthesis of glutathione (which is an antioxidant and DNA (deoxyribonucleic acid).

---

[195] *Overview of Sodium's Role in the Body - Hormonal and Metabolic Disorders.* (n.d.). MSD Manual Consumer Version. https://www.msdmanuals.com/home/hormonal-and-metabolic disorders/electrolyte-balance/overview-of-sodiums-role-in-the-body

You can find magnesium in many natural food options like legumes, whole grains, seeds, and green leafy vegetables.

Phosphorus

Phosphorus is important for the body because it helps build and repair teeth and bones. It also helps in the function of nerves and also in the contraction of muscles.[196] If you do not have a sufficient amount of phosphorus in your body, it can cause diseases in the bone and restriction of bones in children.

Some natural sources of phosphorus are seeds, nuts, poultry products, dairy, meats, beans, and nuts.

Iodine

Iodine holds great importance as they help in the production of thyroid hormones. This is important because it helps in the metabolism of the body and also helps in mental and physical development.

If a child has a deficiency of iodine, it will lead to impaired growth. It also leads to metabolic disorders like goiter. Some mental and menstrual problems also occur due to inadequate levels of iodine.[197] Some women experience problems during pregnancy due to the deficiency of iodine.

One of the easiest sources of iodine is iodized table salt which can be easily available and get your iodine levels sorted.

Iron

This mineral is essential to form hemoglobin. Without hemoglobin, the body could not carry oxygen to the blood

---

[196] MedlinePlus. (2016). *Phosphorus in diet: MedlinePlus medical encyclopedia*. Medlineplus.gov.
https://medlineplus.gov/ency/article/002424.htm

[197] Kapil, U. (2007). Health consequences of iodine deficiency. *Sultan Qaboos University Medical Journal*, 7(3), 267–272.
https://www.ncbi.nlm.nih.gov/pmc/articles/PMC3074887/

effectively. The deficiency of iron can be crucial for the cells of the body and can lead to the death of cells and cellular hypoxia - The oxygen supply is decreased here.

You can get your levels of iron sorted by eating green leafy vegetables. Other than that, meats are also a good source of iron, including pork, chicken, and beef.

Zinc

This mineral is essential for the body as it helps divide cells. Other than that, it also helps to increase the immunity of the body and aids in the healing of wounds. If the levels of zinc are low in the human body, this can cause problems in the immune system.

Some natural sources of zinc are red meat, oysters, beans, poultry, nuts, and whole grains. These provide excellent quantities of zinc and can help in boosting the level of this mineral.

Copper

Copper is considered important due to the production of energy in the body. The body depends on energy for many functions, and coppers help to provide that energy to the body. Other than that, copper also helps absorb iron from the gut, making it essential for the body.

Some dietary sources of copper are liver, chocolate, wheat bran cereals, and shellfish. These are rich in copper and help keep an adequate amount of copper in the body.

Manganese

When you talk about manganese, they are quite important for the human body. This is because they help in the breakdown of carbohydrates as well as cholesterol. It further proceeds to help divide cells, making them vital for the human body. Manganese works with Vitamin K to help in the clotting of blood too. It has a variety of functions in the body. Hence, you must have a sufficient supply of manganese in your body.

Some natural dietary sources of manganese are nuts, whole grains, soybeans, and rice. [198]

Sulfur

Sulfur is a mineral that is enriched with antibacterial properties. Due to these properties, sulfur helps to battle the acne-causing bacteria on the skin. Furthermore, sulfur helps in repairing the damage caused to the DNA. Some of the natural sources of sulfur are legumes like black beans, soybeans, and kidney beans. Seafood is also a rich source of sulfur.

Selenium

This mineral helps prevent oxidative damage caused to the cells. Other than this, selenium is crucial for the metabolism of an important thyroid hormone.[199]

Some natural dietary sources of selenium are seafood, organ meats, and Brazilian nuts.

---

[198] National Institutes of Health. (2017). *Office of Dietary Supplements - Manganese*. Nih.gov. https://ods.od.nih.gov/factsheets/Manganese-HealthProfessional/

[199] Köhrle, J. (2005). Selenium and the Control of Thyroid Hormone Metabolism. *Thyroid*, *15*(8), 841–853. https://doi.org/10.1089/thy.2005.15.841

Importance of Calcium

Calcium is important as it helps perform many basic bodily functions. The body requires calcium for the proper circulation of blood. It also aids in the movement of muscles and helps in the release of hormones. Calcium is deemed important as it is a carrier of messages transmitted from the brain to the other parts of the body. Your tooth and bone health are largely dependent on calcium. Calcium is important as it helps in making the bones stone. The bones are the reservoir of calcium; if the body does not have enough calcium, it will take it from the bones. Hence, it is very important to have sufficient calcium in the body.

The human body does not produce any calcium within itself; hence, getting the needed amount through your diet is important. Some natural foods that are enriched with calcium are dairy products which include cheese, milk, and yogurt. Calcium is also found in green vegetables like spinach, broccoli, and kale. You can get calcium doses from sardines, white beans, and calcium-fortified food like cereals, bread, orange juices, and soy products.

Your body requires Vitamin D to absorb calcium in the body properly.[200] So this means that even if you are taking a diet that has calcium in it, your body will not be able to benefit from it unless there is an adequate amount of Vitamin D in your body.

You can eat foods that are rich in Vitamin D to ensure adequate amounts; these include egg yolks, mushrooms, and salmons. Some products have been added with Vitamin D as well, like milk. You can use them and benefit from Vitamin D.

One amazing source of Vitamin D is sunlight. When your body is exposed to the sun, it encourages the production of Vitamin D in the body through a natural process. You may be

---

[200] NIH. (2018, October). *Calcium and Vitamin D: Important at Every Age | NIH Osteoporosis and Related Bone Diseases National Resource Center.* Nih.gov. https://www.bones.nih.gov/health-info/bone-bone-health/nutrition/calcium-and-vitamin-d-important-every-age

instructed to get Vitamin D supplements so you do not undergo a deficiency of it, as it can also cease calcium absorption.

Women require more calcium than men, and it is considered to be more important for them. It has been researched that PMS symptoms are decreased due to the presence of calcium.

The required amount of calcium in the body depends on the age of human beings. It is recommended that adults should get a thousand milligrams of calcium every single day. Women who are breastfeeding, pregnant, or over the age of 50 should be getting 1,200 mg daily. Having one full cup of skim milk that is low-fat will allow you to get around 300 mg of calcium in your body.

Functions of Calcium

Calcium has many important roles in the body. Without further ado, we are going to discuss these functions.

Calcium Is Essential For Bone Health
Whatever calcium your body gets, 99% of it is reserved for the teeth and the bones. This is because calcium is vital for the development, growth, and also maintenance of the bone.

When a child is in a growing phase, calcium helps develop the bones. After the child stops growing, this mineral becomes important for maintaining the bones. Calcium is responsible for hindering the loss of bone density. The loss of bone density is a natural part of aging.

Women who have gone through menopause can suffer from a loss of bone density at a more accelerated rate than males.[201] This leads to a high chance of osteoporosis. The doctor may be prescribed calcium supplements if required by the body.

Calcium Is Essential For the Contraction of Muscles
Calcium plays an essential role in the contraction of the muscles. When there is a stimulation of nerves in the muscle,

---

[201] Ji, M.-X., & Yu, Q. (2015). Primary osteoporosis in postmenopausal women. *Chronic Diseases and Translational Medicine*, *1*(1), 9–13. https://doi.org/10.1016/j.cdtm.2015.02.006

calcium is released by the body. The calcium that is released aids the proteins that are present in the muscle in contracting. When the calcium is pumped out of the muscle, this will cause the muscles to relax.

Calcium Is Essential For the Clotting Of Blood

Calcium is also important because of the role it plays in the clotting of blood. This process is complicated because it consists of quite a number of steps. Other than that, this process is inclusive of many chemicals, which also include calcium.

Calcium Maintains Activity of the Heart

Calcium helps maintain the activity of the muscle of the heart.[202] This is done by relaxing the smooth muscles that are around the blood vessels. According to the studies, there may be a link between elevated calcium intake and decreased blood pressure.

Calcium Also Has Other Benefits

One of the important roles of calcium is that it behaves as a cofactor for a number of enzymes. Without the presence of calcium in the body, there would be problems with some key enzymes effectively maintaining their work.

Calcium is also important because it has been linked with improvements in the values of cholesterol.[203]

Besides that, calcium is also important because it helps ensure a safe pregnancy by lowering the risk of many conditions like high blood pressure, etc.

Besides, calcium has been seen to lower the risk of a non-cancerous tumor known as colorectal adenomas.

It also helps in lowering blood pressure in young people.

---

[202] Sutanto, H., & Heijman, J. (2019). The role of calcium in the human heart: With great power comes great responsibility. *Frontiers for Young Minds, 7*. https://doi.org/10.3389/frym.2019.00065

[203] Newman, T. (2020, January 28). *Calcium: Health benefits, foods, and deficiency*. Www.medicalnewstoday.com. https://www.medicalnewstoday.com/articles/248958

Signs of Deficiency

Many problems can occur in the human body if there is not an adequate amount of calcium present in it. We will discuss some symptoms that tell us that a person may be suffering from a deficiency of calcium in the body.

Problems in the Muscles
A person who does not have sufficient levels of calcium in the body may experience many muscle problems. Some of them include muscle cramps, muscle spasms, and muscle aches. A person may also feel pain in the arms and thighs, usually because of calcium deficiency. Another problem people face is a tingling or numbness sensation in different parts of their bodies, like arms, hands, legs, feet, and mouth.[204] These symptoms may not stay consistent but may appear often. If a person faces extreme conditions, they can have convulsions, arrhythmias, or even death.

They Face Extreme Fatigue
If a person has low levels of calcium, this can result in them feeling extreme fatigue.[205] This is because of the loss of energy and the lethargic feeling that they have. Also, a deficiency of calcium may lead to insomnia - a person may find it hard to sleep due to the deficiency of calcium.

Along with the deficiency of calcium, a person may experience dizziness, lightheadedness, and brain fog. You can observe it by noticing their confused state of forgetfulness. The deficiency of calcium may even cause people to lack focus.

Problems In the Skin and Nails
If there is a consistent deficiency of calcium in the body, it can be seen through the symptoms occurring in the nails and skin too. You can observe that the skin becomes dry or even suffer from

---

[204] *Numbness and tingling: Causes and treatments.* (2019, August 15). Www.medicalnewstoday.com. https://www.medicalnewstoday.com/articles/326062

[205] Barhum, L. (2020, December 17). *Calcium deficiency disease (hypocalcemia): 7 symptoms and causes.* Www.medicalnewstoday.com. https://www.medicalnewstoday.com/articles/321865

inflammation or eczema; this can result in dry patches along the skin that itch. Psoriasis is a common occurrence in people with a deficiency of calcium.

The nails become brittle and can break easily. You may notice that they are dry and seem quite fragile.[206]

There can be problems in the hair due to the deficiency of calcium. The hair may become coarse, and people have even suffered from alopecia due to calcium deficiency; in this disease, the hair tends to fall out in a bunch.

They Suffer From Osteoporosis and Osteopenia
The bones are the reservoirs of calcium, but adequate amounts of calcium are needed to keep the bones strong and healthy. When the calcium levels in the body are insufficient, it uses the calcium in the bones. This makes the bones brittle and makes them more apt to injury. When you have a reduced amount of calcium in the body for a long time, this can cause osteopenia. Osteopenia is defined as the loss of mineral density in the bones of the body.

If this goes on for a long time, it can result in osteoporosis, where the bones become fragile and are more prone to fractures. People having osteoporosis are usually complaining of pain and problems in their posture. Osteoporosis does not occur overnight and takes a long time to develop.

Severity In PMS
It has been observed that people with lower levels of calcium are related to having severity in the symptoms of (PMS) premenstrual syndrome.

---

[206] *Calcium: Health benefits, foods, and deficiency.* (2020, January 28). Www.medicalnewstoday.com.
https://www.medicalnewstoday.com/articles/248958#takeaway

It Leads to Dental Problems
When the body has a deficiency of calcium, it also uses the calcium from sources like teeth and bones.[207] This may result in many dental problems. People with a reduced calcium level in their body complain of decay in teeth, brittle teeth, weak roots of the tooth, and irritated gums. If an infant does not have a sufficient supply of calcium, it can also hinder the development of the teeth.

It is Linked With Depression
Calcium has been closely monitored to be linked with certain disorders like depression. It is still in the research phase yet and has not been confirmed. Still, people with a calcium deficiency who face depression can talk to their doctors about supplementing calcium.

Signs of Toxicity

The toxicity of calcium can also have a negative impact on the body. One of the symptoms due to the excess calcium can be a pain in the bones and abdomen. It has also been linked to coma and confusion. Elevated levels of calcium can cause a person to go into depression and can also result in diarrhea or constipation.

While we need adequate amounts of calcium, an excess of it can cause loss of appetite, irritability, headache, and irregular heartbeat. It has also been said to cause thirst and weakness in a person. Muscle twitching, vomiting, and nausea are some other symptoms that occur with the toxicity of calcium in the human body.

---

[207] US), M., A Catharine Ross, Taylor, C. L., Yaktine, A. L., & B, H. (2011). *Overview of Calcium*. Nih.gov; National Academies Press (US). https://www.ncbi.nlm.nih.gov/books/NBK56060/

Importance of Chromium

Chromium is an important mineral that is required by the body to carry out its function in a proper way. This mineral occurs in many different forms. Some of the researchers also contradict its benefits of it. One of the damaging forms of chromium can be seen in the pollution caused by industries. The safe form to be used by the body occurs in many natural dietary foods.

The safe form mentioned above is trivalent chromium, which is vital for the body and should be obtained through natural sources.

This mineral is important because it acts as a part of an important molecule known as chromodulin. Chromodulin aids the insulin hormone in effectively completing its role in the body.

The insulin is released by an organ called the pancreas, which helps in processing the body's proteins, fats, and carbs; this is why it is very important for the body.

The chromium is absorbed in very minimal quantity in the intestines; out of all the chromium you intake, less than 2.5% is absorbed by the intestines.[208]

A form of chromium known as chromium picolinate is absorbed in the intestines better; hence, you can find this form in most dietary supplements. The mineral chromium is attached to three molecules of picolinic acid, which makes chromium picolinate - and the body can easily absorb this.

Functions of Chromium

Chromium is important for the body as it performs many functions. Some of the functions are mentioned below:

---

[208] US), M. (2017). *Chromium.* Nih.gov; National Academies Press (US). https://www.ncbi.nlm.nih.gov/books/NBK222329/

Chromium Aids in The Metabolism

Chromium is important because it helps in the metabolism of some macronutrients. These macronutrients include proteins, carbohydrates, and fats/lipids. The chromium makes sure that the complex nutrients are broken down into simpler molecules, and the tissues and cells absorb the nutrients in the body.

Chromium Helps in The Insulin Synthesis

Chromium also acts as a stimulator for the synthesis of insulin.[209] This is done by a mechanism that involves the formation of a bond between an oligopeptide after the ingestion process; this results in the formation of trivalent chromium ions that form a protein known as chromodulin. The chromodulin is responsible for the activation of insulin receptor proteins along with other hormonal functions too.

Chromium Helps in Many Other Functions

Chromium is responsible for promoting the synthesis of cholesterol, which is important for the body; it also helps maintain a balance between the levels of fatty acids found in the human body.

Chromium is responsible for boosting the power of the brain and the nervous systems. This is done by interceding interactions that are done with tissues and neuronal cells.

Another important function of chromium is that it helps strengthen the levels of energy that are required for improved stamina, increased sustenance, and boosted strength of muscles. Other than that, the levels of chromium are also seen to enhance the physical performance of a human being.

Another important function of the human body is that it helps in handling the blood sugar levels of the body and also uplifts the health of the heart.

---

[209] Fu, Z., Gilbert, E. R., & Liu, D. (2013). Regulation of insulin synthesis and secretion and pancreatic Beta-cell dysfunction in diabetes. *Current Diabetes Reviews*, *9*(1), 25–53.
https://www.ncbi.nlm.nih.gov/pmc/articles/PMC3934755/

Signs Of Deficiency

There are several signs of deficiency that can be observed in the human body,

A person may experience a loss of weight due to low levels of chromium. Other than that, it can also confuse them and cause a lapse in coordination. This deficiency can also result in a decreased level of response to the glucose in the bloodstream. This may be sorted with the help of supplements. You may need to consult a healthcare professional for it.

Signs of Toxicity

Consuming high levels of chromium can cause many symptoms.

These are mentioned below:

Fever

Vertigo

Epigastric pain

Vomiting

Diarrhea

Nausea

Ulceration

Cramps in the muscles

Toxic nephritis

Hemorrhagic diathesis

Renal failure

The collapse of the circulatory system

Intravascular hemolysis

Importance of Copper

Copper is considered to be an essential trace mineral that is important for the survival of human beings.[210] This mineral is found in the body tissues and plays an important role in producing red blood cells. Copper is also found in the brain, kidneys, liver, skeletal muscle, and heart. Other than that, this mineral also helps in the maintenance of the immune system and nerve cells. Due to these reasons, it is considered to be very important.

Copper is also important because it helps in the absorption of iron and the formation of collagen.[211] It also plays a crucial role in the production of energy. If you intake too little of an amount of copper, it can affect how your brain works. It can also lead to diseases in the heart. The deficiency of copper is kind of rare.

Functions of Copper

Copper is vital for the human body and is considered an essential nutrient. Working in combination with iron, copper allows the body to produce red blood cells. It also helps in maintaining the health of the bones.

Copper is considered vital for the maintenance of blood vessels, immune functions, and nerves, and it also helps the body in helping with the absorption of iron. It is hinted that an adequate amount of copper in the diet can prevent osteoporosis and cardiovascular disease.

---

[210] Ware, M. (2017, October 23). *Copper: Health benefits, recommended intake, sources, and risks.* Www.medicalnewstoday.com. https://www.medicalnewstoday.com/articles/288165

[211] Ibid.

Copper Helps in Maintaining the Cardiovascular Health of the Body

When there are low levels of copper in the body, it has been linked to a rise in cholesterol and blood pressure.[212] It is recommended by a group of researchers that copper supplements should be given to patients that suffer from the failure of the heart.

According to animal studies, it is seen that low levels of copper lead to cardiovascular diseases. Studies are still going on to clarify if it has the same impact on human beings, too.

Copper Helps in the signaling of Neurons

In 2016, a Professor named Chris Chang designed a fluorescent probe that could detect the movement of copper as it went in and out of nerve cells. According to Prof. Chang, copper acts as a dimmer for brake for each one of the nerve cells.

Copper Improves the Immune Function of the Body

If your body does not have adequate amounts of copper, it can lead to neutropenia. [213]The body goes through a deficiency of neutrophils or white blood cells in neutropenia, which fights off the infection.

Copper Reduces the Risk of Osteoporosis

A severe deficiency of copper can lead to a lower bone mineral density, bringing a higher risk of osteoporosis. There is a need for more research to prove that the deficiency of copper can lead to problems in the health of the bone, and it can also be linked to copper supplements being a solution to this problem.

---

[212] DiNicolantonio, J. J., Mangan, D., & O'Keefe, J. H. (2018). Copper deficiency may be a leading cause of ischaemic heart disease. *Open Heart*, 5(2), e000784. https://doi.org/10.1136/openhrt-2018-000784

[213] Ware, M. (2017, October 23). *Copper: Health benefits, recommended intake, sources, and risks*. Www.medicalnewstoday.com. https://www.medicalnewstoday.com/articles/288165

Copper Maintains the Production of Collagen
According to the hypothesis of many scientists, it is believed that copper plays an important role in maintaining the levels of elastin and collagen in the body. These serve as the structural segments of the human body. According to a hypothesis, it is also believed that copper has antioxidant properties, which prevent skin aging.

Copper Deficiency can Lead to Arthritis
According to studies on animals, it is seen that the presence of copper may help in delaying or even preventing arthritis. This is the reason that many people also wear copper bracelets - though no human studies are known to confirm this.

Copper May Act as an Antioxidant
Copper is also thought to act as an antioxidant; due to this, it helps in the reduction of the production of free radicals. It also has several other functions, like producing the red blood cells of the body. It also helps to regulate the blood pressure and the heart rate of the body. Other than that, it helps absorb the iron in the human body and also helps to prevent prostatitis. Copper is also essential for maintaining and developing the bone, heart, brain, and connective tissues.

Signs of Deficiency

If a human has a deficiency of copper in the body, it can be shown through anemia and low body temperature symptoms.[214] Other symptoms include the onset of osteoporosis and a low count of white blood cells. It will be shown on the skin through the loss of pigment and can result in thyroid problems. Another symptom of copper deficiency is an irregular heartbeat.

Signs of Toxicity

Some symptoms are telltales of the toxicity of copper too. These include frequent headaches and passing out for no apparent

---

[214] Raman, R. (2018). *9 Signs and Symptoms of Copper Deficiency*. Healthline. https://www.healthline.com/nutrition/copper-deficiency-symptoms

reason. People can also have a fever or feel sick, or vomit due to the toxicity of copper. Often the vomiting is seen to have blood in it too. People with copper toxicity also have reported black poop, diarrhea, and abdominal cramps. In certain cases, people with access to copper had brown ring-shaped markings in the eyes known as Kayser-Fleischer rings. It can also cause the yellowing of skin and eyes.

Importance of Fluoride

Fluoride is a mineral that is required for the teeth and bones of the human body. This mineral is found naturally in plants, air, soils, water, and rocks.

This mineral is often used to make the enamel of the teeth strong. Enamel is known as the layer which is present outside the teeth. [215]Due to fluoride, cavities are prevented. Fluoride is also added to public water in many countries, and this process is termed water fluoridation.

Fluoride is used for many things, including the improvement of dental health. Fluoride is included in many over-the-counter products, including supplements, toothpaste, and mouth rinses.

If a person gets a lot of cavities, they may be advised to rinse their mouth with fluoride. Fluoride is also used for medical imaging scans that include PET scans. It can also be used in pesticides and as a cleaning agent.

Functions of Fluoride

Some functions of fluoride include the following;

1. It remineralizes the tooth enamel that had been weakened. [216]
2. It helps in reversing the early signs of tooth decay.
3. It also helps in slowing down the mineral loss from the enamel of the tooth.
4. It helps in the prevention of the growth of toxic oral bacteria.

---

[215] *Teeth are Made of THESE Three Layers | Asleep For Dentistry.* (2019). Asleepfordentistry.com. http://www.asleepfordentistry.com/blog/three-layers-of-a-tooth.html

[216] *Dental Remineralization: Simplified.* (n.d.). Oral Health Group. Retrieved December 16, 2022, from https://www.oralhealthgroup.com/features/dental-remineralization-simplified/

Signs of Deficiency

The deficiency of fluoride can be observed in a weakness in the bones and teeth.

In the human body, fluoride is mainly contained in the teeth and bones.[217] Adequate amounts of fluoride are necessary to ensure the health of teeth and bones.

Signs of Toxicity

If fluoride is toxic in the human body, this can be observed through the following symptoms:

- Diarrhea
- Drooling
- Irregular heartbeat
- Slow heartbeat
- Abnormal levels of calcium in the blood
- Abnormal levels of potassium in the blood
- Irritation in the eyes
- Abdominal pain
- Headache
- Strange taste in the mouth

---

[217] *Office of Dietary Supplements - Fluoride.* (n.d.). Ods.od.nih.gov. https://ods.od.nih.gov/factsheets/Fluoride-HealthProfessional/

Importance of Iron

The maintenance of healthy blood in the body is done due to an important mineral known as iron. When there is a deficiency of iron, it is termed iron-deficiency anemia, and this affects 4-5 million Americans every year.

Amongst all, iron deficiency is one of the most common nutritional deficiencies that take place globally, and this causes lightheadedness and severe fatigue in the body. This deficiency is not restricted to any particular age or gender and can occur in any age, in men or women, including women who are menstruating or pregnant. People who have to receive dialysis for kidneys are also at a very high risk of this deficiency.

Iron is a significant constituent of hemoglobin, a protein found in RBCs (Red Blood Cells), and can carry oxygen from the lungs to all the different body parts. [218] When there is not an adequate amount of iron in the body, there will not be a sufficient amount of red blood cells for the transportation of oxygen, too - this will lead to fatigue in the human body.

Apart from hemoglobin, iron also constitutes a part of myoglobin; this protein transports oxygen to muscles and helps in the storage of it too. Iron is crucial for the healthy development of the brain and proper growth in children, and it also helps in the proper function and production of many different hormones and cells.

When you consume food with iron, it comes in two forms: non-heme and heme. When we talk about heme, it is mainly found in animal flesh like seafood, poultry, and meat. Where non-heme is considered, it can be found in nuts, legumes, whole grains, seeds, and leafy greens. You can also find non-heme iron in the flesh of animals; this is because the animals tend to ingest plant foods that

---

[218] UCSF Health. (2019, March 14). *Hemoglobin and Functions of Iron.* Ucsfhealth.org; UCSF Health.
https://www.ucsfhealth.org/education/hemoglobin-and-functions-of-iron

are stacked with non-heme iron and foods that are fortified with it too.

Iron is stored in the muscle tissue, kicker, bone marrow, and spleen in the form of ferritin. A protein known as transferrin is used to transport this throughout the body; this protein is found in blood and can bind to iron. The doctor may prescribe tests for the presence of transferrin and ferritin in the blood of humans.

In adults that are of 19-50 years of age, 18 mg is the Recommended Dietary Allowance for females, while 8 mg is the RDA for men. If the woman is pregnant, 27 mg is the Recommended Dietary Allowance, while 9 mg is for lactating mothers. Women require more iron as they lose blood when they are menstruating. [219] Also, during pregnancy, the growth of the fetus requires an additional circulation of blood. Adolescents aged 14-18 and in a growing phase also require a higher amount of iron - the girls require 15 mg, while the boys require 11 mg.

When the women are 50 plus age, the Recommended Dietary Allowance drops to 8 mg; this is because menstruation usually stops at that point, and hence the blood loss is discontinued. If menopause is delayed, you can always consult the healthcare professional about following the Recommended Dietary Allowance for younger women.

The Upper Intake Level (UL) of iron for each day is 45 mg - this goes for all males and females who exceed the age of 14 years. For children who are under the age of 14 have a UL of 40 mg.

Functions of Iron

Iron is known to perform many functions in the body. These functions are mentioned below.

---

[219] Harvey, L. J., Armah, C. N., Dainty, J. R., Foxall, R. J., Lewis, D. J., Langford, N. J., & Fairweather-Tait, S. J. (2005). Impact of menstrual blood loss and diet on iron deficiency among women in the UK. *British Journal of Nutrition*, 94(4), 557–564. https://doi.org/10.1079/bjn20051493

Iron Is Essential For The Process Of Cell Division

In order for the process of mitosis to take place in the body, iron is needed. Mitosis is a process that occurs as a segment of the cell cycle. [220] Here, the cells are divided in such a way that it gives rise to identical cells bearing the same amount of chromosomes.

Mitosis consists of five different stages. The first is called prophase, then prometaphase, metaphase, anaphase, and telophase.

During mitosis, the duplicated chromosomes tend to act on fibers that help get one copy of each chromosome on the opposite sides of the cell.

Iron Helps in Reducing Fatigue and Tiredness in Humans

According to a study conducted, it was seen that the ladies who took the supplements of iron faced 48% lesser fatigue than those women who did not take any supplements.[221]

This study explains the importance of iron, especially for pregnant women or athletes who require more energy to function better.

Iron is essential for the cognitive function of the body

Iron is vital for the cognitive functions of the body, and this includes problem-solving abilities, memory, learning, and concentration. It will boost your brain if there are adequate quantities of iron in the system. If you drink coffee to enhance your ability to concentrate, you would not require it if you have enough iron in your body.

---

[220] Khan Academy. (2015). *Phases of mitosis*. Khan Academy. https://www.khanacademy.org/science/ap-biology/cell-communication-and-cell-cycle/cell-cycle/a/phases-of-mitosis

[221] Yilma, H., Sedlander, E., Rimal, R. N., & Pattnaik, S. (2020). Is fatigue a cue to obtain iron supplements in Odisha, India? A mixed methods investigation. *BMJ Open, 10*(10), e037471. https://doi.org/10.1136/bmjopen-2020-037471

Iron helps in performing functions of the immune system
You can observe a link between the immune system and iron. Iron is a key mineral in the body that helps create cells and also helps in their growth. Also, iron plays a vital role in the health of the immune system because of its requirement for the proliferation and maturation of the immune cells. The lymphocytes also require iron, which is closely linked to your body's response to infections.

Iron helps the body in the production of energy
Iron is important for the body because it is one of the most vital minerals that is required. Human beings get their energy from food iron is needed by the cells to convert food into energy. The more iron you have in your body, the more energy you can get. However, if you have an excessive amount of iron in your body, it can also be a source of some health issues. So, it is better to keep it in a specified range.

Iron helps in the transportation of oxygen in the body
One of the most crucial functions of iron is that it can transport oxygen to the blood. Moreover, the main purpose of iron is to transport oxygen by carrying it in the hemoglobin of the RBCs (Red Blood Cells) and circulating it in your entire body so that the cells can produce energy. Other than that, iron is helpful for the improvement of the storage of oxygen through myoglobin. Myoglobin is a protein that contains iron and initiates the transport and storage of oxygen in the muscles.

Iron helps in the production of red blood cells and hemoglobin
Iron is also used for the synthesis of heme which helps in the formation of hemoglobin - a protein that is present in the RBCs (Red Blood Cells).[222] Hemoglobin is responsible for the transportation of oxygen between the lungs and the tissues of the body; this helps in the maintenance of the basic functions of life performed by the human body. If this process does not occur, the

---

[222] Sciences, N. A. of S. (US) and N. R. C. (US) D. of M. (1958). THE ROLE OF IRON IN HEMOGLOBIN SYNTHESIS. In *www.ncbi.nlm.nih.gov*. National Academies Press (US).
https://www.ncbi.nlm.nih.gov/books/NBK224286/

body will be unable to regulate enough oxygen, and you will be exhausted.

Signs of Deficiency

In the beginning, the symptoms of iron deficiency anemia are quite mild. People are not even able to notice them in the initial part. Until a blood test is done, people do not even realize they have mild anemia.

A person with a moderate or severe deficiency of iron can be noticed due to the following symptoms.

The person can complain of fatigue and weakness. They may feel shortness of breath and even have pale skin. Some people are impacted by dizziness, while others feel a weird craving that compels them to eat things with no nutritional value.

Some symptoms are a crawling or a tingling sensation in the legs or soreness or swelling in the tongue. Iron deficiency can also be characterized by cold feet and hands and often irregular or fast heartbeat.[223] People also experience brittle nails and headaches when they have iron deficiency.

Iron deficiency is the most common cause of anemia, and people may get deficient for many reasons.

Pregnancy or Menstruation

When women are pregnant or lose blood through the process of menstruation, they can go through iron deficiency anemia. During pregnancy, the human body requires more iron as it also generates oxygen for the baby.[224]

Insufficient Intake of Iron

If your consumption of iron-rich foods is low for a long period of time, it can lead to a deficiency of iron in the body. You can eat foods that have iron in them like eggs, green leafy vegetables, and

---

[223] Mayo Clinic. (2019, October 18). *Iron deficiency anemia - Symptoms and causes*. Mayo Clinic; Mayo Clinic. https://www.mayoclinic.org/diseases-conditions/iron-deficiency-anemia/symptoms-causes/syc-20355034

[224] Institute of Medicine (US) Committee on Nutritional Status During Pregnancy and Lactation. (2016). *Iron Nutrition During Pregnancy*. Nih.gov; National Academies Press (US). https://www.ncbi.nlm.nih.gov/books/NBK235217/

meat. Iron is very important for the development and growth of the fetus and young children; hence, younger ones and pregnant women should ensure to eat an iron-rich diet.

Internal Bleeding

Certain conditions can cause internal bleeding that can lead to iron deficiency anemia. Some examples of these conditions are ulcers in the stomach, polyps that occur in the intestine or colon, and colon cancer. A regular intake of pain relievers can also lead to stomach bleeding.

Endometriosis

You may be unaware of the presence of endometriosis because it hides in the pelvic or abdominal area outside the uterus. A person with endometriosis may have heavy blood loss during their menstrual periods. This can also be the cause of iron deficiency in many women.

The Inability of the Body to Absorb Iron

Certain disorders of the body and surgeries can impact the intestines and interfere with their ability to absorb iron; due to this, even when you consume a diet rich in iron, the absorption of it is limited.[225]

Genetics

Genetics can also play a part in the absorption of iron. [226]Some conditions, for instance, celiac disease, make it hard for iron to be absorbed in the human body. This disease is passed on to the family through genetics and can also be enhanced by mutations like the TMRPSS mutation. Due to this mutation, the body absorbs lots of hepcidin. The absorption of hepcidin would prevent a blockage of the intestines from absorbing any iron.

---

[225] Saboor, M. (1969). Disorders associated with malabsorption of iron; a critical review. *Pakistan Journal of Medical Sciences, 31*(6). https://doi.org/10.12669/pjms.316.8125

[226] *Iron Absorption - an overview | ScienceDirect Topics.* (n.d.). Www.sciencedirect.com. Retrieved December 28, 2022, from https://www.sciencedirect.com/topics/biochemistry-genetics-and-molecular-biology/iron-absorption

There are other conditions related to genetics that can cause anemia too. This can be done by abnormal bleeding, too; hemophilia and Von Willebrand diseases are examples of it.

Signs of Toxicity

If there is iron toxicity in the body, the person may show some symptoms like seizures, yellowing of the skin (jaundice), or bluish-grayish skin color. Some people might even suffer from low blood pressure or an elevated or weak pulse. Headache, dizziness, and fever are more characteristics of elevated levels of iron in the body. A person may even go through shortness of breath due to iron toxicity.

Importance of Iodine

Iodine is a mineral used mainly by the thyroid.[227] Human beings are incapable of making iodine on their own. Hence it is supposed to be ingested through food. Iodine is added to the salt and foods too.

Iodine can keep the thyroid hormone in perfect working condition and kill bacteria, amoebas, and fungus. The deficiency of iodine is one of the world's most common nutritional problems. Mostly, iodine can be found in the ocean, as it is condensed by sea life, specifically seaweed.

Iodine can be ingested through the diet to avoid its deficiency. Iron deficiency possesses a lot of consequences, like thyroid disorders and goiter. A US FDA-approved potassium iodide is used to prevent damage to the thyroid after radioactive events. Iodine can also relieve gum infections and heal wounds and pink eye; there is only a little scientific evidence that supports this, though.

Functions of Iodine

Iodine is an essential mineral for the body. It is needed by the body, especially during pregnancy; this is because the exposure of iodine to the fetus may help prevent health risks later in life. Here are a few uses of iodine in the human body.

It Helps In the Promotion of the Thyroid Health
Iodine is essential for the health of the thyroid. The thyroid gland is placed at the base of the front part of the human neck.[228]

---

[227] Zelman, K. (2015). *Iodine a Critically Important Nutrient*. Eatright.org. https://www.eatright.org/food/vitamins-and-supplements/types-of-vitamins-and-nutrients/iodine-a-critically-important-nutrient

[228] Society for Endocrinology. (2018, March). *Thyroid gland | You and Your Hormones from the Society for Endocrinology*. Yourhormones.info. https://www.yourhormones.info/glands/thyroid-gland/

This gland regulates the production of hormones that help deal with heart health, metabolism, etc.

The body requires iodine in small amounts to create thyroid hormones. If there is an insufficient supply of iodine in the body, the production of the hormones might be altered. An underactive thyroid gland can give rise to a condition known as hypothyroidism.

Iodine is widely available in many dishes globally. Hence the low levels do not usually occur due to the absence of it. You can get iodine by ingesting fortified foods, salt water, fish, and dairy products. Iodine can also be found in plant foods that are grown in soil that is rich in iodine. Iodized salt is another important source of iodine for the human body.

While your body does require iodine, excess of it is also bad for the body and causes a negative impact. Hence, it is recommended that you do not take iodine supplements till you consult your healthcare professional.

It Helps in Reducing the Risk of Certain Goiters

A goiter is a condition in which the thyroid gland becomes enlarged. The thyroid can become enlarged due to hyperthyroidism or hypothyroidism. When a person suffers from hyperthyroidism, they have an overactive thyroid gland.

When there is a presence of non–cancerous thyroid nodules, this can also give rise to thyroid enlargement. There are times when the goiter can even be caused due to a deficiency of iodine. The goiters that are induced by the absence of iodine are reversible by consuming an iodine-rich diet and iodine supplements.

It Helps In Managing an Overactive Thyroid Gland

When there is an overactive thyroid gland, your doctor may prescribe a specific type of iodine to help deal with that condition.[229] This iodine is called radioiodine and is consumed as

---

[229] Cleveland Clinic. (2021). *Hyperthyroidism: Symptoms, Causes, and Treatment & Medication.* Cleveland Clinic. https://my.clevelandclinic.org/health/diseases/14129-hyperthyroidism

a medication. It helps in the destruction of the thyroid's extra cells, which aids in the reduction of excessive thyroid hormone.

There is always a risk with this radioactive iodine that it may cause a larger amount of thyroid cells than needed; this can also cause hypothyroidism in the body. Due to this reason, radioactive iodine is recommended only if the anti-thyroid drugs stop responding. Be sure you understand that radioactive and iodine supplements are two entirely separate things.

Radioiodine is also a treatment option for thyroid cancer.[230] It is based on the same mechanism as with the treatment of hyperthyroidism. The medication is used to destroy thyroid cells, including cancerous cells. It is often given after thyroid surgery to destroy the remains of the cancerous cells from the body.

It is seen that radioiodine medications are good at improving the rate of survival in people with thyroid cancer.

It Helps In the Improvement of the Cognitive Function
Iodine can benefit the neurological functions of the human body. It can make the brain function healthy. Hence, the presence of iodine can reduce the risk of intellectual disability in humans. If your child is getting a sufficient amount of iodine through their diet, yet you feel worried about their iodine intake, then you must talk to their pediatrician.

It Helps In the Development of the Nervous System during Pregnancy
You require more iodine during pregnancy; this is because iodine intake during pregnancy can help in the development of the brain in the fetus.[231] According to research, mothers who had an iodine deficiency during the time of pregnancy were said to have

---

[230] American Cancer Society. (2019, March 14). *Radioactive Iodine (Radioiodine) Therapy for Thyroid Cancer*. Cancer.org; American Cancer Society. https://www.cancer.org/cancer/thyroid-cancer/treating/radioactive-iodine.html

[231] *Vol 11 Issue 12 p.5-6*. (n.d.). American Thyroid Association. https://www.thyroid.org/patient-thyroid-information/ct-for-patients/december-2018/vol-11-issue-12-p-5-6/

children with a lower IQ as well as a hindrance in other intellectual activities.

A woman who is pregnant can always talk to their healthcare professional about the addition of iodine supplements. If you are generally deficient in that mineral, there may also be a requirement for iodine supplements. Breastfeeding women may even require to monitor their iodine levels. The iodine you take in your supplements and diet is also transferred to the infant through breast milk.

It Helps In Improving the Birth Weight
During pregnancy, Iodine helps develop the brain and is also related to healthy birth weight. It was observed that in pregnant women who had goiters, 400 mg of iodine helped alter their goiter condition. Along with that, it was observed that there was an improvement in the newborn babies of all the women. This study was linked to women who were deficient in iodine and iron.

It is vital that you do not take iodine supplements till you are prescribed by your healthcare professional.

Signs of Deficiency

If a person has a deficiency of iodine, it can usually be noticed by the swelling in the front of the neck; this is one of the biggest symptoms of iodine deficiency. When the thyroid gland becomes enlarged, this condition is known as goiter.

Other than that, people also gain weight due to the deficiency of iodine. This happens because the body has insufficient iodine to form thyroid hormones. The thyroid hormones help in speeding up the process of metabolism. Other than this, thyroid hormones also help control the growth of hair follicles. With lower iodine, the thyroid hormones would be lesser, which can cause your hair follicles to cease the process of regeneration.

People with lower iodine in their systems tend to feel colder than they usually do and may even notice changes in their heart rate. Other than that, people with low iodine and low thyroid hormones may feel weak sluggish, and fatigued.

Signs of Toxicity

If there is an excess of iodine in the human body, there may be abdominal pain and delirium. Other symptoms include coughing and a metallic taste in the mouth. People may lose their appetite and also feel a soreness in the tooth or gums. Apart from this, the symptoms of iodine toxicity also include diarrhea, which can also be bloody, and fever.[232]

---

[232] *Iodine poisoning Information | Mount Sinai - New York.* (n.d.). Mount Sinai Health System. https://www.mountsinai.org/health-library/poison/iodine-poisoning

Importance of Magnesium

Magnesium is important for the body as it helps in muscle support, energy production, and nerve function. Low magnesium levels in the human body can cause an increased risk of high blood pressure. It can also increase the risk of type 2 diabetes, osteoporosis, and even heart disease.

Magnesium is important because it plays an active role in around three hundred enzymatic reactions in the human body.

Functions of Magnesium

Magnesium plays a lot of roles in the human body.

It Helps In the Creation of Energy
Magnesium is important because it helps in the conversion of food into energy.

It Helps In the Maintenance of Genes
Magnesium is crucial for the body because of its role in creating and repairing RNA and DNA.

It Helps In the Formation of Proteins
The Magnesium in the body helps in the creation of amino acids and new proteins.

It Helps In Regulating the Nervous System
Magnesium plays a significant role in the regulation of neurotransmitters in the body. These neurotransmitters are responsible for the transport of messages in the nervous system and brain.

It May Help In Battling Depression
A person with lower levels of Magnesium is often linked with depression. [233]

---

[233] Tarleton, E. K., & Littenberg, B. (2015). Magnesium intake and depression in adults. *Journal of the American Board of Family Medicine: JABFM, 28*(2), 249–256. https://doi.org/10.3122/jabfm.2015.02.140176

Signs of Deficiency

A deficiency of Magnesium can cause the following symptoms in the human body.

It promotes a loss of appetite and therefore leads to weakness and fatigue. People can also suffer from shaking, nausea and vomiting. There are cases where low levels of Magnesium have been linked with abnormal heart rhythms, muscle spasms, or even sleepiness. Some people might even experience pins and needles or hyper-excitability.

Signs of Toxicity

The toxicity of Magnesium usually occurs when the concentration of the serum is raised to 1.74-2.61 mmol/L.[234]

When this happens, a person can feel nauseated and suffer from hypotension. Some people feel like vomiting or depressed. There can be flushing of the face or the retention of urine due to the toxicity of Magnesium. Some people may even have difficulty breathing, muscle weakness, or irregular heartbeat.

---

[234] *Office of Dietary Supplements - Magnesium.* (2013). Nih.gov. https://ods.od.nih.gov/factsheets/Magnesium-HealthProfessional%20/

Importance of Manganese

Manganese is an important mineral found in many foods like seeds, tea, legumes, nuts, leafy green vegetables, and whole grains. The human body requires it because it helps the body to function properly. Manganese is also used by the people as a form of medicine. It is widely used for osteoarthritis and osteoporosis - brittle and weak bones. Moreover, it is required for other conditions as well.

Functions of Manganese

Manganese has a couple of functions in the human body.

It Helps Produce Enzymes
Manganese is important for the body because it helps the body in producing a variety of enzymes and also antioxidants. These help in battling against free radical damage and also aids in the metabolism of lipids and carbohydrates.

It Boosts the Important Systems of The Body
Manganese is considered to be very important for the function of the brain and a healthy nervous system.

It Helps In Dealing with Arthritis
The supplements of manganese are also used in treating the problems of arthritis in people. They also help in the betterment of the conditions of osteoporosis. The supplements of manganese are often merged with chondroitin and glucosamine. Hence the sole effects of manganese on arthritis and osteoporosis are still not proven. It helps in the proper formation of bones and gives them strength.

It May Help People With Diabetes
Most of the time, it has been seen that people suffering from diabetes are usually suggested Magnese supplements.[235] It is observed that manganese plays an important role in glucose metabolism, though it is not observed yet.

It Helps In the Metabolism
Your body also contains many enzymes that help speed up chemical reactions. Being a necessary component of many important enzymes, manganese works to process cholesterol, carbohydrates, and amino acids.

It Has Antioxidant Properties
It is an antioxidant and hence helps stop the free radicals that damage your body's cells. The main detoxifier of free radicals is manganese-containing enzymes.

Signs of Deficiency

The deficiency of manganese can lead to many problems, like skeletal defects and poor growth of bone. It can also lead to impaired or slow growth. Other than that, manganese deficiency can even cause low fertility and abnormal carbohydrate and fat metabolism.

Apart from that, deficiency of manganese is also linked with an impaired glucose tolerance which is a state that resides between normal metabolism of glucose and diabetes.

Signs of Toxicity

The toxicity of manganese can be dangerous as it can lead to a neurological disorder with permanent effects - this is known as manganism.

---

[235] *Manganese – Health Information Library | PeaceHealth.* (n.d.). Www.peacehealth.org. Retrieved December 28, 2022, from https://www.peacehealth.org/medical-topics/id/hn-2881000

The manganism symptoms include difficulty walking, spasms in the muscles of the face, and tremors. [236]

These symptoms usually occur after the lesser intensive symptoms like aggressiveness, irritable mood, and a tendency to hallucinate.

---

[236] *Manganism - an overview | ScienceDirect Topics*. (n.d.). Www.sciencedirect.com. Retrieved December 28, 2022, from https://www.sciencedirect.com/topics/nursing-and-health-professions/manganism

Importance of Molybdenum

Like Magnesium and Iron, Molybdenum is also known as an important mineral in the human body. It is present in the soil, so getting it into your diet may seem a bit confusing. Well, you can get Molybdenum through the plants that are present in that molybdenum-enriched soil. Also, you can get the Molybdenum from the animals that ingest the plants growing in that soil.

The amounts of Molybdenum may vary considerably in these, but in usual cases, the best sources of it are beans, organs, meats like kidney and liver, meats, grains, and lentils. There are many other poor sources of Molybdenum, too. These include other animal products, vegetables, and fruits.

According to the studies, the human body does not absorb Molybdenum from some products, including soy ones. But this is not much of a problem as other foods are rich in this mineral. The human body requires only some trace amounts of Molybdenum, and they are found in abundance in man foods; due to this factor, the deficiency of Molybdenum is seen to be quite low. Due to this, people do not even need many supplements for this particular mineral.

Functions of Molybdenum

Molybdenum is quite important for the human body. When a human ingests Molybdenum, it is essential for the processes of the body. Once you ingest the food with this mineral in it, it gets absorbed into your gut and stomach through the blood. It is then transported to the kidneys, liver, and also other areas.

The livers and kidneys store some of the minerals, but the maximum amount of it undergoes conversion to the molybdenum cofactor. Any excess Molybdenum in the body is passed out by the body through the process of urination.

Signs of Deficiency

Molybdenum deficiency is generally rare because human beings get it from a wide variety of food.[237] Hence supplements of Molybdenum are not commonly used either. The deficiency of Molybdenum can cause a decrease in libido. Other symptoms include the reduction of spermatogenesis and may even result in sterility in males.

The deficiency of Molybdenum can also delay puberty in children and reduces the rate of conception and anestrus in women.

Signs of Toxicity

The toxicity of this mineral is often due to the increase of copper-molybdenum in the body of humans. [238]The people who undergo this can show symptoms like infertility and poor growth. Some people also show signs of diarrhea, osteoporosis, and ataxia due to the toxicity of this mineral.

---

[237] Institute of Medicine (US) Panel on Micronutrients. (2015). *Molybdenum*. Nih.gov; National Academies Press (US).
https://www.ncbi.nlm.nih.gov/books/NBK222301/
[238] Ibid.

Importance of Phosphorus

Phosphorus is a mineral that is present in many different foods and can also be found as a supplement. It helps in performing many roles in the body of humans. It is important as it is a key element for cell membranes, teeth, and bones. Other than that, it also helps in the activation of enzymes and enables the blood pH to stay within limits.

Phosphorus helps in the regulation of the functions performed by the muscles, heart, and nerves. It also acts as a building block of many genes and helps in making the structure of RNA, DNA, and ATP- which is the most significant source of energy in the body.

The bones, intestines, and kidneys all help in the regulation of phosphorus in the human body. If there is a lack of phosphorous in the diet of humans, there are mechanisms that take place to help in the storage of the phosphorus and maintain the required levels; for instance, the kidney would start excreting lesser amounts of phosphorus in the urine while the digestive system would work more efficiently to absorb the phosphorus. The bones also help in releasing the stored amount of phosphorus in the blood. If the body has a sufficient amount of phosphorus in it, then the systems would work in just the opposite ways to maintain the balance of phosphorus in the body.

Functions of Phosphorus

It Helps In Strengthen the Teeth
Phosphorus is one of those minerals that is found in abundance in the body. Around 85% of the phosphorus is stored in the teeth and the bones. It works with calcium to keep the teeth and bones healthy.

It Helps In the Production of Energy
Phosphorus helps our body in the production of energy and also aids in keeping the pH balance in the body.

It Helps In the Formation of Genetic Material

Phosphorus helps in the production of the genetic material that is RNA and DNA.[239] Other than that, it also helps in the transportation of oxygen through the RBCs (Red Blood Cells) of the body. Other than that, phosphorus is also responsible for the production of phospholipids.

Signs of Deficiency

The condition when there is a deficiency of phosphorus in the body is known as hypophosphatemia. This happens when the level of phosphorus gets too low in the blood, and this can also cause a lack of energy in the body. Other than that, some symptoms of the deficiency of phosphorus are fatigue, low exercise tolerance, and also muscle weakness.

The inadequate levels of phosphorus, along with the low levels of vitamin D and calcium, can lead to the softening and weakening of bones - this usually takes a long time to happen. This also causes pain in the muscles and joints.

Signs of Toxicity

If there is an excessive quantity of phosphorus in the body, the human body may show some symptoms like muscle weakness and pains, joint pain, and also can cause red eyes and itching.

Some people can also suffer from diarrhea, nausea, constipation, and vomiting.

---

[239] Arnarson, A. (2017, May 24). *20 Foods That Are High in Vitamin E*. Healthline. https://www.healthline.com/nutrition/foods-high-in-vitamin-e

Importance of Selenium

Selenium is important in the human body because it helps maintain the thyroid hormone. Besides that, this mineral is crucial for synthesizing DNA and protects the body from oxidative infection and damage.

Selenium is stored in the tissues of humans and can be mostly found in the skeletal muscles.[240] The food containing selenium in them are meats, Brazilian nuts, and also, seafood.

The selenium in the food depends on the soil and water concentration of the place where it grew. This mineral is also added to the food or can also be ingested in the form of supplements.

Functions of Selenium

Selenium is known for its many functions in the human body.

It Behaves As an Antioxidant
When the process of metabolism takes place in the body, the free radicals are usually the byproducts in such a case. They have regularly formed in the body. When you smoke or use alcohol, this can cause an excessive amount of these free radicals in the body. Selenium is a powerful antioxidant and battles against these free radicals and the world to protect the body.

It Protects Against the Heart Disease
A selenium-rich diet helps to maintain the heart and keeps it healthy. When humans have a low amount of selenium in their bodies, it is often linked with an increased risk of certain heart diseases.

---

[240] *15 high selenium foods: Why we need them, and more.* (2021, May 5). Www.medicalnewstoday.com.
https://www.medicalnewstoday.com/articles/foods-with-selenium#summary

It May Reduce the Chances of Some Cancers
Selenium reduces the risk of certain cancers in the human body. This happens through the destruction of the cancerous cells.

It Helps In Preventing the Decline of Mental Abilities
Alzheimer's disease is a mental disease that causes the loss of memory and also harms the behavior and thinking of people. According to research, it is known as the 6th leading reason of death in the United States of America.

Oxidative stress is linked with the initiation of Alzheimer's and Parkinson's disease. [241] It also helps oxidative battle stress and hinders the decline of mental health.

Signs of Deficiency

If a human body has an inadequate supply of selenium, it will start to show signs like a foggy mental state and weakness of the muscles. People even experience fatigue and can get a weakened immune system too. Other cases have even shown symptoms of the loss of hair and infertility.

Signs of Toxicity

If the body has an extra level of selenium, it shows signs like discoloration in the nails and brittleness. Other signs are linked to vomiting, hair loss, fatigue, bad breath, irritable mood, and nausea.

---

[241] Pimentel, C., Batista-Nascimento, L., Rodrigues-Pousada, C., & Menezes, R. A. (2012). Oxidative stress in Alzheimer's and Parkinson's diseases: insights from the yeast Saccharomyces cerevisiae. *Oxidative Medicine and Cellular Longevity*, *2012*, 132146. https://doi.org/10.1155/2012/132146

Importance of Potassium

This is an important mineral that comes under the classification of an electrolyte. This is because the mineral is very reactive in the water. When you dissolve potassium in water, it ends up with the production of positively charged ions. Due to this, the conduction of electricity can be done, which is quite important for actively running many processes in the body of humans.

When your diet is rich in potassium, you can get many health benefits too. This is because adequate levels of potassium help in maintaining blood pressure and balance water retention. Other than that, the presence of a sufficient amount of potassium is also linked with protection against stroke and may also help prevent stones in the kidney and osteoporosis.

The third most abundant mineral that is present in the body is potassium.[242] It also helps in sending nerve signals and regulating the contraction of muscles. When you notice the presence of potassium, you will observe that around 98% of the cells are present in the cells of the body. 80% are located in the cells of the muscles, while the remaining ones are located in the red blood cells, bones, and liver.

When it is in the body of humans, this starts to function as an electrolyte. When placed in the water, the electrolyte completely dissolves and forms negative and positive ions that possess the ability to conduct electricity. The ions of the potassium are positively charged.

This electricity is used by the body to manage many different processes like the contraction of the muscles, signaling of the nerves, and also fluid balance.

---

[242] Raman, R. (2017). *What Does Potassium Do for Your Body? A Detailed Review*. Healthline.
https://www.healthline.com/nutrition/what-does-potassium-do

Functions of Potassium

It Helps In the Regulation of Fluid Balance
Sixty percent of the human body is made with water, and forty percent of the water is located in the cells in a substance and is known as ICF - Intracellular fluid. The remaining water is found in the cells that are outside the cells, like the spinal fluid, blood, and also in between the cells of the body. This fluid is known as ECF - Extracellular fluid.

The amount of water that is present in the ICF and ECF is deeply affected by the potassium and sodium concentrations. Potassium holds the place of utmost importance as the electrolyte in the ICG and also helps in determining the water amount that is present in the cells.

In contrast, sodium secures the position as the main electrolyte that is present in the ECF and helps in determining the presence of the water amount that is located outside the cells. [243]

Thus, potassium is very important for the regulation of fluid balance.

It Is Important For the Nervous System
The nervous system holds works to transmit messages between the brain and the body. This is done with the help of nerve impulses, which also help in the contraction of muscles, reflexes, and also the heartbeat. The nerve impulses are also generated by the potassium making its way out of the cells and sodium ions making their way into the cells.

It Helps In the Regulation of Heart and Muscle Contractions
The potassium levels also affect the regulation of muscle and heart contractions. This is done by the effect of nerve signals that take

---

[243] Tobias, A., & Mohiuddin, S. S. (2020). *Physiology, Water Balance.* PubMed; StatPearls Publishing.
https://www.ncbi.nlm.nih.gov/books/NBK541059/

place on the nervous system - these weaken the contractions of the muscles.

Signs of Deficiency

Potassium, when in insufficient quantity in the body, can show signs like tiredness, muscle cramps, and weakness. It can also lead to constipation and confusion. Potassium deficiency has also been linked to an increase in urination, numbness or tingling, and also arrhythmia - an unsteady rhythm of the heart.

Signs of Toxicity

People with an excess of potassium in their bodies may show signs like diarrhea and abdominal pain. [244]It can also cause arrhythmia or palpitations in the heart. Chest pain, numbness in limbs, and weakness in the muscles can also take place due to the toxicity of potassium. Some people also feel like vomiting or suffer from nausea due to potassium toxicity.

---

[244] Cleveland Clinic. (2016). *Hyperkalemia and Potassium Levels | Cleveland Clinic*. Cleveland Clinic. https://my.clevelandclinic.org/health/diseases/15184-hyperkalemia-high-blood-potassium

Importance of Zinc

Zinc is a mineral that is needed in very minute quantities by the body. While it is needed in trace quantities, it is still required by hundred of enzymes to go through their vital chemical reactions. This is a major player that aids in the growth of the cells, DNA creation, protein building, and healing of the damaged tissues. It also helps to support the immune system and keeps it healthy.

For this, you require zinc in your diet, and it can be ingested through a wide range of animal and plant sources.

Functions of Zinc

It Accelerates the Healing Of the Wounds
This mineral is apt in its role in the synthesis of collagen, and hence it is required for the proper healing of wounds. [245]It also helps in strengthening the inflammatory response and immune function of the body.

It May Help In Battling a Couple of Diseases
Zinc is known to decrease the risk of many diseases that are related to age, like infections, age-related macular degeneration, and pneumonia. It may help in relieving oxidative stress, which can help in the improvement of the immune response. This can also help in protecting the body of humans from infection.

It Helps In Boosting the Immune System
Zinc is known to keep the immune system strong and healthy. If there is an inadequate level of zinc, this can lead to a weak response of the immune system.

---

[245] Eat Well Nutrition Service. (2021). *Nutrition and Wound Healing | Eat Well Nutrition*. Eat Well Nutrition.
https://www.eatwellnutrition.com.au/wound-healing/nutrition-and-wound-healing

Signs of Deficiency

The deficiency of zinc in the body can show signs like retardation in growth, impaired immune function, and also appetite loss. [246]Other than that, a deficiency of zinc can also lead to a loss of hair, delay in sexual maturation, diarrhea, hypogonadism (males), impotence, and lesions in the skin and eye.

Signs of Toxicity

Excessive levels of zinc are linked with vomiting and nausea, diarrhea, and a change in taste. People can also experience flu-like symptoms and go through frequent infections.

---

[246] Hassan, A., Sada, K.-K., Ketheeswaran, S., Dubey, A. K., & Bhat, M. S. (2020). Role of Zinc in Mucosal Health and Disease: A Review of Physiological, Biochemical, and Molecular Processes. *Cureus*, *12*(5). https://doi.org/10.7759/cureus.8197

Bibliography

"The 10 Best Foods High in Vitamin E." *Medical News Today*, MediLexicon International, https://www.medicalnewstoday.com/articles/324308#.

"The 10 Best Foods High in Vitamin E." *Medical News Today*, MediLexicon International, https://www.medicalnewstoday.com/articles/324308#peanuts.

14 Iron Nutrition during Pregnancy - NCBI Bookshelf. https://www.ncbi.nlm.nih.gov/books/NBK235217/.

2 Overview of Calcium - NCBI Bookshelf. https://www.ncbi.nlm.nih.gov/books/NBK56060/.

"9 Biotin-Rich Foods to Add to Your Diet." *Medical News Today*, MediLexicon International, https://www.medicalnewstoday.com/articles/320222.

"9 Biotin-Rich Foods to Add to Your Diet." *Medical News Today*, MediLexicon International, https://www.medicalnewstoday.com/articles/320222.

AC, Ross, et al. *2 Overview of Calcium - NCBI Bookshelf.* https://www.ncbi.nlm.nih.gov/books/NBK56060/.

Alaei Shahmiri F;Soares MJ;Zhao Y;Sherriff J; "High-Dose Thiamine Supplementation Improves Glucose Tolerance in Hyperglycemic Individuals: A Randomized, Double-Blind Cross-over Trial." *European Journal of Nutrition*, U.S. National Library of Medicine, https://pubmed.ncbi.nlm.nih.gov/23715873/.

Alisi, Ludovico, et al. "The Relationships between Vitamin K and Cognition: A Review of Current Evidence." *Frontiers in Neurology*, Frontiers Media S.A., 19 Mar. 2019, https://www.ncbi.nlm.nih.gov/pmc/articles/PMC6436180/.

Alma, Lori. "What Is the Difference between Fat-Soluble and Water-Soluble Vitamins?" *Verywell Health*, Verywell Health, 19 Aug. 2021, https://www.verywellhealth.com/fat-vs-water-soluble-998218.

Amber, Ann-Mary. "Riboflavin Diet: How to Age Less: Look Great: Live Longer: Health and Lifestyle." *Slow Aging | Healthy Living, Healthy Aging*, 20 Jan. 2018, https://slowaging.org/vitamin-b2-and-aging/.

The American Cancer Society medical and editorial content team. "Radioactive Iodine (Radioiodine) Therapy for Thyroid Cancer." *American Cancer Society*, https://www.cancer.org/cancer/thyroid-cancer/treating/radioactive-iodine.html.

Andrews, Nancy C. "Iron Absorption." *Iron Absorption - an Overview | ScienceDirect Topics*, https://www.sciencedirect.com/topics/biochemistry-genetics-and-molecular-biology/iron-absorption.

"Antioxidants." *Antioxidants - Better Health Channel*, https://www.betterhealth.vic.gov.au/health/healthyliving/antioxidants.

Anwar, Adnan, et al. "Thiamine Level in Type I and Type II Diabetes Mellitus Patients: A Comparative Study Focusing on Hematological and Biochemical Evaluations." *Cureus*, Cureus, 8 May 2020, https://www.ncbi.nlm.nih.gov/pmc/articles/PMC7282352/.

Ao, Misora, et al. "Possible Involvement of Thiamine Insufficiency in Heart Failure in the Institutionalized Elderly." *Journal of Clinical Biochemistry and Nutrition*,

The Society for Free Radical Research Japan, May 2019, https://www.ncbi.nlm.nih.gov/pmc/articles/PMC6529701/.

"Are Sardines Good for You? Nutritional Benefits and More." *Medical News Today*, MediLexicon International, https://www.medicalnewstoday.com/articles/are-sardines-good-for-you.

Authors Ana Spasojevic, et al. "The Role of Calcium in the Human Heart: With Great Power Comes Great Responsibility." *Frontiers for Young Minds*, https://kids.frontiersin.org/articles/10.3389/frym.2019.00065.

Baswan, Sudhir M., et al. *Application of Sunscreen – Theory and Reality - Wiley Online Library*. 5 May 2021, https://onlinelibrary.wiley.com/doi/full/10.1111/phpp.12099.

Bennet, John E. "Enzymes." *Enzymes - an Overview | ScienceDirect Topics*, https://www.sciencedirect.com/topics/neuroscience/enzymes.

Berkheiser, Kaitlyn. "9 Health Benefits of Vitamin B12, Based on Science." *Healthline*, Healthline Media, 14 June 2018, https://www.healthline.com/nutrition/vitamin-b12-benefits.

"Beta-Carotene." *Mount Sinai Health System*, https://www.mountsinai.org/health-library/supplement/beta-carotene#:~:text=Dietary%20Sources,more%20beta%2Dcarotene%20it%20has.

"Big Doses of Vitamin C May Lower Blood Pressure - 04/18/2012." *Johns Hopkins Medicine, Based in Baltimore, Maryland*, https://www.hopkinsmedicine.org/news/media/releases/big_doses_of_vitamin_c_may_lower_blood_pressure.

"Big Doses of Vitamin C May Lower Blood Pressure - 04/18/2012." *Johns Hopkins Medicine, Based in Baltimore, Maryland*, https://www.hopkinsmedicine.org/news/media/releases/big_doses_of_vitamin_c_may_lower_blood_pressure.

"Big Doses of Vitamin C May Lower Blood Pressure - 04/18/2012." *Johns Hopkins Medicine, Based in Baltimore, Maryland*, https://www.hopkinsmedicine.org/news/media/releases/big_doses_of_vitamin_c_may_lower_blood_pressure.

"Biotin (Vitamin B7) for Hair Growth: Uses, Sources, Health Benefits." *Medical News Today*, MediLexicon International, https://www.medicalnewstoday.com/articles/287720.

"Biotin (Vitamin B7) for Hair Growth: Uses, Sources, Health Benefits." *Medical News Today*, MediLexicon International, https://www.medicalnewstoday.com/articles/287720.

"The Blood Clotting Process: What Happens If You Have a Bleeding Disorder." *HemAware*, 24 July 2020, https://hemaware.org/bleeding-disorders-z/blood-clotting-process-what-happens-if-you-have-bleeding-disorder.

Brazier, Yvette. "Vitamin B2: Role, Sources, and Deficiency." *Medical News Today*, MediLexicon International, https://www.medicalnewstoday.com/articles/219561.

Brazier, Yvette. "Vitamins: What Are They, and What Do They Do?" *Medical News Today*, MediLexicon International, 15 Dec. 2020, https://www.medicalnewstoday.com/articles/195878.

Brennan, Dan. "8 Foods High in Niacin and Why You Need Ityo." *WebMD*, WebMD, 3 Nov. 2020, https://www.webmd.com/diet/foods-high-in-niacin-b3#1.

"Broccoli: Health Benefits, Nutrition, and Tips." *Medical News Today*, MediLexicon International, https://www.medicalnewstoday.com/articles/266765.

BSc, Atli Arnarson. "20 Foods That Are High in Vitamin E." *Healthline*, Healthline Media, 24 May 2017, https://www.healthline.com/nutrition/foods-high-in-vitamin-e.

BSc, Atli Arnarson. "20 Foods That Are High in Vitamin E." *Healthline*, Healthline Media, 24 May 2017, https://www.healthline.com/nutrition/foods-high-in-vitamin-e.

BSc, Atli Arnarson. "20 Foods That Are High in Vitamin E." *Healthline*, Healthline Media, 24 May 2017, https://www.healthline.com/nutrition/foods-high-in-vitamin-e.

BSc, Atli Arnarson. "20 Foods That Are High in Vitamin E." *Healthline*, Healthline Media, 24 May 2017, https://www.healthline.com/nutrition/foods-high-in-vitamin-e.

BSc, Atli Arnarson. "Corn 101: Nutrition Facts and Health Benefits." *Healthline*, Healthline Media, 16 May 2019, https://www.healthline.com/nutrition/foods/corn.

BSc, Atli Arnarson. "The Fat-Soluble Vitamins." *Healthline*, Healthline Media, 16 Feb. 2017, https://www.healthline.com/nutrition/fat-soluble-vitamins#:~:text=Vitamins%20can%20be%20classified%20based,do%20not%20dissolve%20in%20water.

Cabrera-Rode E;Molina G;Arranz C;Vera M;González P;Suárez R;Prieto M;Padrón S;León R;Tillan J;García I;Tiberti

C;Rodríguez OM;Gutiérrez A;Fernández T;Govea A;Hernández J;Chiong D;Domínguez E;Di Mario U;Díaz-Díaz O;Díaz-Horta O; "Effect of Standard Nicotinamide in the Prevention of Type 1 Diabetes in First Degree Relatives of Persons with Type 1 Diabetes." *Autoimmunity*, U.S. National Library of Medicine, https://pubmed.ncbi.nlm.nih.gov/16891222/.

Caito, Samuel, and Michael Aschner. "Manganism." *Manganism - an Overview | ScienceDirect Topics*, 2015, https://www.sciencedirect.com/topics/nursing-and-health-professions/manganism.

"Calcitonin: What It Is, Function & Side Effects." *Cleveland Clinic*, https://my.clevelandclinic.org/health/articles/22330-calcitonin.

"Calcitonin: What It Is, Function & Side Effects." *Cleveland Clinic*, https://my.clevelandclinic.org/health/articles/22330-calcitonin.

"Calcium and Bones: Medlineplus Medical Encyclopedia." *MedlinePlus*, U.S. National Library of Medicine, https://medlineplus.gov/ency/article/002062.htm.

"Calcium and Vitamin D: Important at Every Age." *National Institutes of Health*, U.S. Department of Health and Human Services, https://www.bones.nih.gov/health-info/bone/bone-health/nutrition/calcium-and-vitamin-d-important-every-age.

"Calcium Deficiency and Nails: Link, Signs, Treatment, and More." *Medical News Today*, MediLexicon International, https://www.medicalnewstoday.com/articles/calcium-deficiency-nails.

"Calcium Deficiency Disease (Hypocalcemia): 7 Symptoms and Causes." *Medical News Today*, MediLexicon International, https://www.medicalnewstoday.com/articles/321865.

"Calcium: Health Benefits, Foods, and Deficiency." *Medical News Today*, MediLexicon International, https://www.medicalnewstoday.com/articles/248958.

Calderón-Ospina, Carlos Alberto, and Mauricio Orlando Nava-Mesa. "B Vitamins in the Nervous System: Current Knowledge of the Biochemical Modes of Action and Synergies of Thiamine, Pyridoxine, and Cobalamin." *CNS Neuroscience & Therapeutics*, John Wiley and Sons Inc., Jan. 2020, https://www.ncbi.nlm.nih.gov/pmc/articles/PMC6930825/.

Center for Food Safety and Applied Nutrition. "Questions and Answers on Dietary Supplements." *U.S. Food and Drug Administration*, FDA, https://www.fda.gov/food/information-consumers-using-dietary-supplements/questions-and-answers-dietary-supplements.

Chadwick, Melanie Rud. "Dermatologists Want You to Use Panthenol with Your Hyaluronic Acid Products." *Byrdie*, Byrdie, 27 Apr. 2022, https://www.byrdie.com/panthenol-for-skin-the-complete-guide-4770218.

Chambial, Shailja, et al. "Vitamin C in Disease Prevention and Cure: An Overview." *Indian Journal of Clinical Biochemistry : IJCB*, Springer India, Oct. 2013, https://www.ncbi.nlm.nih.gov/pmc/articles/PMC3783921/.

Cherney, Kristeen. "Niacinamide: 10 Benefits for Skin, Topical or Supplement, Side Effects." *Healthline*, Healthline

Media, 29 Aug. 2018, https://www.healthline.com/health/beauty-skin-care/niacinamide.

"Circulatory System." *Circulatory System - Better Health Channel*, https://www.betterhealth.vic.gov.au/health/conditionsandtreatments/circulatory-system.

Clifford , J., and A. Kozil. "Fat-Soluble Vitamins: A, D, E, and K - 9.315." *Extension*, 27 Mar. 2019, https://extension.colostate.edu/topic-areas/nutrition-food-safety-health/fat-soluble-vitamins-a-d-e-and-k-9-315/.

Clifford, J., and A. Kozil. "Fat-Soluble Vitamins: A, D, E, and K - 9.315 - Extension." *Fat-Soluble Vitamins: A, D, E, and K – 9.315* , https://extension.colostate.edu/topic-areas/nutrition-food-safety-health/fat-soluble-vitamins-a-d-e-and-k-9-315/.

Contributors, WebMD Editorial. "Beta Carotene: Health Benefits, Safety Information, Dosage, and More." *WebMD*, WebMD, https://www.webmd.com/diet/health-benefits-beta-carotene.

Contributors, WebMD Editorial. "Vitamin B1 (Thiamine): Foods and Health Benefits." *WebMD*, WebMD, https://www.webmd.com/vitamins-and-supplements/health-benefits-of-vitamin-b-1.

Contributors, WebMD Editorial. "Vitamin B1 (Thiamine): Foods and Health Benefits." *WebMD*, WebMD, https://www.webmd.com/vitamins-and-supplements/health-benefits-of-vitamin-b-1.

Coyle, Daisy. "Top 7 Health Benefits of Asparagus." *Healthline*, Healthline Media, 4 Apr. 2018, https://www.healthline.com/nutrition/asparagus-benefits.

"Depression, Aggression, and Vitamin B1 Thiamine Supplements as a New Treatment." *Eat2BeNice*, 15 May 2020, https://newbrainnutrition.com/depression-aggression-and-vitamin-b1-thiamine-supplements-as-a-new-treatment/.

"Did You Know That Hot Chilli Peppers Have More Vitamin C than Oranges? Health Benefits of the Popular Spice." *Latest News by Times Now News*, https://www.timesnownews.com/health/article/did-you-know-that-hot-chilli-peppers-have-more-vitamin-c-than-oranges-health-benefits-of-the-popular-spice/654351.

Dix, Megan. "Oxidative Stress: Definition, Effects on the Body, and Prevention." *Healthline*, Healthline Media, 29 Sept. 2018, https://www.healthline.com/health/oxidative-stress.

Dix, Megan. "Pellagra: Pictures, Symptoms, Causes, and Treatment." *Healthline*, Healthline Media, 18 Sept. 2018, https://www.healthline.com/health/pellagra.

"Dysmenorrhea: What It Is, Treatments, Causes." *Cleveland Clinic*, https://my.clevelandclinic.org/health/diseases/4148-dysmenorrhea.

Fast Facts Fat Soluble Vitamins 063015 - University of Washington. https://depts.washington.edu/ceeh/downloads/Fast%20Facts%20Fat%20Soluble%20Vitamins%20063015.pdf.

Fast Facts Fat Soluble Vitamins 063015 - University of Washington. https://depts.washington.edu/ceeh/downloads/Fast%20Facts%20Fat%20Soluble%20Vitamins%20063015.pdf.

FINCH, CLEMENT A. "Home - Books - NCBI." *National Center for Biotechnology Information*, U.S. National

Library of Medicine, https://www.ncbi.nlm.nih.gov/books.

Fletcher, Jenna. "Fat-Soluble Vitamins: Types, Function, and Sources." *Medical News Today*, MediLexicon International, 17 Jan. 2020, https://www.medicalnewstoday.com/articles/320310.

"Folate (Folic Acid) – Vitamin B9." *The Nutrition Source*, 2 July 2019, https://www.hsph.harvard.edu/nutritionsource/folic-acid/.

"Folate (Folic Acid) – Vitamin B9." *The Nutrition Source*, 2 July 2019, https://www.hsph.harvard.edu/nutritionsource/folic-acid/.

"Folate (Folic Acid) – Vitamin B9." *The Nutrition Source*, 2 July 2019, https://www.hsph.harvard.edu/nutritionsource/folic-acid/.

"Folate (Folic Acid) – Vitamin B9." *The Nutrition Source*, 2 July 2019, https://www.hsph.harvard.edu/nutritionsource/folic-acid/.

"Folic Acid and Pregnancy (for Parents) - Nemours Kidshealth." Edited by Thinh Phu Nguyen, *KidsHealth*, The Nemours Foundation, July 2022, https://kidshealth.org/en/parents/preg-folic-acid.html.

"Folic Acid Helps Prevent Some Birth Defects." *Centers for Disease Control and Prevention*, Centers for Disease Control and Prevention, 17 June 2022, https://www.cdc.gov/ncbddd/folicacid/features/folic-acid-helps-prevent-some-birth-defects.html.

"Folic Acid." *Centers for Disease Control and Prevention*, Centers for Disease Control and Prevention, 17 Nov. 2020, https://www.cdc.gov/ncbddd/folicacid/index.html.

Fu, Zhuo, et al. "Regulation of Insulin Synthesis and Secretion and Pancreatic Beta-Cell Dysfunction in Diabetes." *Current Diabetes Reviews*, U.S. National Library of Medicine, 1 Jan. 2013, https://www.ncbi.nlm.nih.gov/pmc/articles/PMC3934755/.

Goldstep, Fay. "Dental Remineralization: Simplified." *Oral Health Group*, 3 June 2016, https://www.oralhealthgroup.com/features/dental-remineralization-simplified/#.

Gunnars, Kris. "10 Health Benefits of Kale." *Healthline*, Healthline Media, 29 June 2018, https://www.healthline.com/nutrition/10-proven-benefits-of-kale.

Gunnars, Kris. "Spinach 101: Nutrition Facts and Health Benefits." *Healthline*, Healthline Media, 14 May 2019, https://www.healthline.com/nutrition/foods/spinach.

H;, McGarel C;Pentieva K;Strain JJ;McNulty. "Emerging Roles for Folate and Related B-Vitamins in Brain Health across the Lifecycle." *The Proceedings of the Nutrition Society*, U.S. National Library of Medicine, https://pubmed.ncbi.nlm.nih.gov/25371067/.

Harvey LJ;Armah CN;Dainty JR;Foxall RJ;John Lewis D;Langford NJ;Fairweather-Tait SJ; "Impact of Menstrual Blood Loss and Diet on Iron Deficiency among Women in the UK." *The British Journal of Nutrition*, U.S. National Library of Medicine, https://pubmed.ncbi.nlm.nih.gov/16197581/.

Hassan, Abbas, et al. "Role of Zinc in Mucosal Health and Disease: A Review of Physiological, Biochemical, and Molecular Processes." *Cureus*, Cureus, 19 May 2020, https://www.ncbi.nlm.nih.gov/pmc/articles/PMC7302722/.

Hassan, Abbas, et al. "Role of Zinc in Mucosal Health and Disease: A Review of Physiological, Biochemical, and Molecular Processes." *Cureus*, Cureus, 19 May 2020, https://www.ncbi.nlm.nih.gov/pmc/articles/PMC7302722/.

Helpguidewp. "Vitamins and Minerals." *HelpGuide.org*, 8 Feb. 2022, https://www.helpguide.org/harvard/vitamins-and-minerals.htm.

"Home - Books - NCBI." *National Center for Biotechnology Information*, U.S. National Library of Medicine, https://www.ncbi.nlm.nih.gov/books.

"Home - Books - NCBI." *National Center for Biotechnology Information*, U.S. National Library of Medicine, https://www.ncbi.nlm.nih.gov/books.

"Home - Books - NCBI." *National Center for Biotechnology Information*, U.S. National Library of Medicine, https://www.ncbi.nlm.nih.gov/books.

"Home." *You and Your Hormones*, https://www.yourhormones.info/glands/thyroid-gland/.

"Home." *You and Your Hormones*, https://www.yourhormones.info/hormones/vitamin-d/.

"Homocysteine Test: Medlineplus Medical Test." *MedlinePlus*, U.S. National Library of Medicine, https://medlineplus.gov/lab-tests/homocysteine-test/.

"Homocysteine: Levels, Tests, High Homocysteine Levels." *Cleveland Clinic*, https://my.clevelandclinic.org/health/articles/21527-homocysteine.

"Hyperkalemia (High Blood Potassium): Symptoms, Causes & Treatment." *Cleveland Clinic*, https://my.clevelandclinic.org/health/diseases/15184-hyperkalemia-high-blood-potassium.

"Hyperthyroidism: Symptoms, Causes, Treatment & Medication." *Cleveland Clinic*, https://my.clevelandclinic.org/health/diseases/14129-hyperthyroidism.

III, James L. Lewis. "Overview of Sodium's Role in the Body - Hormonal and Metabolic Disorders." *MSD Manual Consumer Version*, MSD Manuals, 4 Aug. 2022, https://www.msdmanuals.com/home/hormonal-and-metabolic-disorders/electrolyte-balance/overview-of-sodiums-role-in-the-body.

"Iodine Poisoning." *Mount Sinai Health System*, https://www.mountsinai.org/health-library/poison/iodine-poisoning.

"Iron in Diet: Medlineplus Medical Encyclopedia." *MedlinePlus*, U.S. National Library of Medicine, https://medlineplus.gov/ency/article/002422.htm.

Is It a Mineral - University of Nevada, Reno. https://nbmg.unr.edu/_docs/ScienceEducation/Activities/WhatIsAMineral.pdf.

"Is It Better to Get Nutrients from Food or Supplements?" *Medical News Today*, MediLexicon International, https://www.medicalnewstoday.com/articles/324956.

J;, Köhrle. "Selenium and the Control of Thyroid Hormone Metabolism." *Thyroid : Official Journal of the American Thyroid Association*, U.S. National Library of Medicine, https://pubmed.ncbi.nlm.nih.gov/16131327/.

Jayne Leonard. "9 Biotin-Rich Foods to Add to Your Diet." *Medical News Today*, MediLexicon International, https://www.medicalnewstoday.com/articles/320222.

Jennings, Kerri-Ann. "Pumpkin: Nutrition, Benefits, and How to Eat It." *Healthline*, Healthline Media, 9 Sept. 2021, https://www.healthline.com/nutrition/pumpkin-nutrition-review#.

Ji, Meng-Xia, and Qi Yu. "Primary Osteoporosis in Postmenopausal Women." *Chronic Diseases and Translational Medicine*, KeAi Publishing, 21 Mar. 2015, https://www.ncbi.nlm.nih.gov/pmc/articles/PMC5643776/.

Johnson, Jon. "9 Ways to Stimulate Collagen Production in Skin." *Medical News Today*, MediLexicon International, https://www.medicalnewstoday.com/articles/317151.

Johnson, Larry E. "Vitamin B6 Deficiency - Disorders of Nutrition." *MSD Manual Consumer Version*, MSD Manuals, 4 Aug. 2022, https://www.msdmanuals.com/home/disorders-of-nutrition/vitamins/vitamin-b6-deficiency.

Julson, Erica. "16 Foods That Are High in Niacin (Vitamin B3)." *Healthline*, Healthline Media, 5 Oct. 2018, https://www.healthline.com/nutrition/foods-high-in-niacin.

Julson, Erica. "16 Foods That Are High in Niacin (Vitamin B3)." *Healthline*, Healthline Media, 5 Oct. 2018, https://www.healthline.com/nutrition/foods-high-in-niacin.

Julson, Erica. "16 Foods That Are High in Niacin (Vitamin B3)." *Healthline*, Healthline Media, 5 Oct. 2018, https://www.healthline.com/nutrition/foods-high-in-niacin.

K;, El-Akawi Z;Abdel-Latif N;Abdul-Razzak. "Does the Plasma Level of Vitamins A and E Affect Acne Condition?" *Clinical and Experimental Dermatology*, U.S. National

Library of Medicine, https://pubmed.ncbi.nlm.nih.gov/16681594/.

Kannan, Rajendran, and Matthew Joo Ming Ng. "Cutaneous Lesions and Vitamin B12 Deficiency: An Often-Forgotten Link." *Canadian Family Physician Medecin De Famille Canadien*, College of Family Physicians of Canada, Apr. 2008, https://www.ncbi.nlm.nih.gov/pmc/articles/PMC2294086/.

Kannan, Rajendran, and Matthew Joo Ming Ng. "Cutaneous Lesions and Vitamin B12 Deficiency: An Often-Forgotten Link." *Canadian Family Physician Medecin De Famille Canadien*, College of Family Physicians of Canada, Apr. 2008, https://www.ncbi.nlm.nih.gov/pmc/articles/PMC2294086/.

Kapil, Umesh. "Health Consequences of Iodine Deficiency." *Sultan Qaboos University Medical Journal*, Sultan Qaboos University Medical Journal, College of Medicine & Health Sciences, Dec. 2007, https://www.ncbi.nlm.nih.gov/pmc/articles/PMC3074887/.

Kelly, Steve. "Is Beef Liver Good or Bad for You?" *Heartstone Farm*, Heartstone Farm, 19 Mar. 2019, https://www.heartstonefarm.me/blogs/about-grass-fed-beef/is-beef-liver-good-or-bad-for-you.

Khazaei, Hamid, et al. "Seed Protein of Lentils: Current Status, Progress, and Food Applications." *Foods (Basel, Switzerland)*, MDPI, 4 Sept. 2019, https://www.ncbi.nlm.nih.gov/pmc/articles/PMC6769807/.

Kheiri, Babikir, et al. "Vitamin D Deficiency and Risk of Cardiovascular Diseases: A Narrative Review." *Clinical*

Hypertension, BioMed Central, 22 June 2018, https://www.ncbi.nlm.nih.gov/pmc/articles/PMC6013996/.

Kubala, Jillian. "7 Benefits of Eating Avocados, According to a Dietitian." *Healthline*, Healthline Media, 29 June 2022, https://www.healthline.com/nutrition/avocado-nutrition.

Lacey, Jennifer. "Pregnancy B Vitamins: How Important Are They?" *Healthline*, Healthline Media, 3 Sept. 2015, https://www.healthline.com/health/pregnancy/b-vitamins.

Lauren Wicks   Lauren Wicks   Reviewed by Dietitian Lisa Valente, M.S. "4 Amazing Health Benefits of Sunflower Seeds." *EatingWell*, https://www.eatingwell.com/article/2059940/sunflower-seeds-nutrition/.

Leech, Joe. "11 Evidence-Based Health Benefits of Eating Fish." *Healthline*, Healthline Media, 11 June 2019, https://www.healthline.com/nutrition/11-health-benefits-of-fish.

Leech, Joe. "9 Evidence-Based Health Benefits of Almonds." *Healthline*, Healthline Media, 6 Sept. 2018, https://www.healthline.com/nutrition/9-proven-benefits-of-almonds.

Leech, Joe. "Legumes: Good or Bad?" *Healthline*, Healthline Media, 29 July 2019, https://www.healthline.com/nutrition/legumes-good-or-bad.

Leech, Joe. "Vitamin K2." *Healthline*, Healthline Media, 11 May 2022, https://www.healthline.com/nutrition/vitamin-k2.

Leoni Jesner, ACE-CPT. "Why Vitamin B Complex Is Important to Your Health." *Verywell Fit*, https://www.verywellfit.com/b-complex-vitamins-89411.

Libretexts. "6.3: Vitamins Important for Metabolism." *Medicine LibreTexts*, Libretexts, 14 Aug. 2020, https://med.libretexts.org/Courses/American_Public_University/APUS%3A_An_Introduction_to_Nutrition_(Byerley)/APUS%3A_An_Introduction_to_Nutrition_1st_Edition/06%3A_Energy_Metabolism/6.03%3A_Vitamins_Important_for_Metabolism#:~:text=Key%20Takeaways-,Vitamins%20and%20minerals%20play%20a%20different%20kind%20of%20role%20in,protein%2C%20RNA%2C%20and%20DNA.

Link, Rachael. "15 Healthy Foods That Are High in Folate (Folic Acid)." *Healthline*, Healthline Media, 27 Feb. 2020, https://www.healthline.com/nutrition/foods-high-in-folate-folic-acid.

Link, Rachael. "5 Surprising Health Benefits of Orange Juice." *Healthline*, Healthline Media, 12 Feb. 2019, https://www.healthline.com/nutrition/orange-juice-benefits.

"List of Foods That Are High in Vitamin C." *Which Foods Are High In Vitamin C – Health Insurance Blog By Reliance General*, Reliance General Insurance Home Page, https://www.reliancegeneral.co.in/Insurance/Knowledge-Center/Blogs/List-Of-Foods-That-Are-High-In-Vitamin-C.aspx.

"Listing of Vitamins." *Harvard Health*, 31 Aug. 2020, https://www.health.harvard.edu/staying-healthy/listing_of_vitamins.

Lykstad , J, and S. Sharma. "Home - Books - NCBI." *National Center for Biotechnology Information*, U.S. National Library of Medicine, Jan. 2022, https://www.ncbi.nlm.nih.gov/books.

Lykstad, Jacqueline, and Sandeep Sharma. "National Center for Biotechnology Information." *Biochemistry, Water*

Soluble Vitamins, StatPearls Publishing LLC, Jan. 2022, https://www.ncbi.nlm.nih.gov/books/NBK538510/.

"Macular Degeneration (AMD): Symptoms, Causes, Treatment, Prevention." *WebMD*, WebMD, https://www.webmd.com/eye-health/macular-degeneration/age-related-macular-degeneration-overview#:~:text=Age%2Drelated%20macular%20degeneration%20(AMD,called%20the%20macula%2C%20wears%20down.

"Manganese." *PeaceHealth*, https://www.peacehealth.org/medical-topics/id/hn-2881000.

Mann, P. J. G., and J. H. Quastel. "Vitamin B1 and Acetylcholine Formation in Isolated Brain." *Nature News*, Nature Publishing Group, https://www.nature.com/articles/145856a0.

McCulloch, Marsha. "15 Healthy Foods High in B Vitamins." *Healthline*, Healthline Media, 11 Oct. 2018, https://www.healthline.com/nutrition/vitamin-b-foods.

"The Mechanism for Vitamin A Improvements in Night Vision." Edited by Anthony J. Busti, *EBM Consult*, https://www.ebmconsult.com/articles/vitamin-a-eye-vision-mechanism.

"Medical Definition of Vitamin B2." Edited by Charles Patrick Davis, *RxList*, RxList, 29 Mar. 2021, https://www.rxlist.com/vitamin_b2/definition.htm.

Megaloblastic Anemia - Statpearls - NCBI Bookshelf. https://www.ncbi.nlm.nih.gov/books/NBK537254/.

Moore, Marisa. "How Vitamin C Supports a Healthy Immune System." *EatRight*, https://www.eatright.org/food/vitamins-and-supplements/types-of-vitamins-and-nutrients/how-vitamin-c-supports-a-healthy-immune-system.

Morris, Rebecca. "Vitamin B5 (Pantothenic Acid)." *Healthline*, Healthline Media, 15 Aug. 2018, https://www.healthline.com/health/vitamin-watch-what-does-b5-do.

National Center for Biotechnology Information. https://www.ncbi.nlm.nih.gov/books/NBK234926/.

National Center for Biotechnology Information. https://www.ncbi.nlm.nih.gov/books/NBK234926/.

National Center for Biotechnology Information. https://www.ncbi.nlm.nih.gov/books/NBK538510/.

NCBI Bookshelf. https://www.ncbi.nlm.nih.gov/books/NBK541059/.

"NCI Dictionary of Cancer Terms." *National Cancer Institute*, https://www.cancer.gov/publications/dictionaries/cancer-terms/def/vitamin-b-complex.

"Niacin to Improve Cholesterol Numbers." *Mayo Clinic*, Mayo Foundation for Medical Education and Research, 7 June 2022, https://www.mayoclinic.org/diseases-conditions/high-blood-cholesterol/in-depth/niacin/art-20046208.

"Numbness and Tingling: Causes and Treatments." *Medical News Today*, MediLexicon International, https://www.medicalnewstoday.com/articles/326062.

Nutrition, Food Safety & Health - Extension. https://extension.colostate.edu/topic-areas/nutrition-food-safety-health/.

"Nutrition, Food Safety & Health." *Extension*, 11 Apr. 2022, https://extension.colostate.edu/topic-areas/nutrition-food-safety-health/.

"Office of Dietary Supplements - Fluoride." *NIH Office of Dietary Supplements*, U.S. Department of Health and Human Services, https://ods.od.nih.gov/factsheets/Fluoride-HealthProfessional/.

"Office of Dietary Supplements - Magnesium." *NIH Office of Dietary Supplements*, U.S. Department of Health and Human Services, https://ods.od.nih.gov/factsheets/Magnesium-HealthProfessional%20/.

"Office of Dietary Supplements - Manganese." *NIH Office of Dietary Supplements*, U.S. Department of Health and Human Services, https://ods.od.nih.gov/factsheets/Manganese-HealthProfessional/.

"Office of Dietary Supplements - Thiamin." *NIH Office of Dietary Supplements*, U.S. Department of Health and Human Services, https://ods.od.nih.gov/factsheets/Thiamin-HealthProfessional/.

"Office of Dietary Supplements - Vitamin B6." *NIH Office of Dietary Supplements*, U.S. Department of Health and Human Services, https://ods.od.nih.gov/factsheets/VitaminB6-HealthProfessional/.

"Office of Dietary Supplements - Vitamin B6." *NIH Office of Dietary Supplements*, U.S. Department of Health and Human Services, https://ods.od.nih.gov/factsheets/VitaminB6-HealthProfessional/.

Olsen, Natalie. "Benefits of Beta Carotene and How to Get It." *Healthline*, Healthline Media, 13 Aug. 2020, https://www.healthline.com/health/beta-carotene-benefits#:~:text=Diets%20rich%20in%20carotenoids%20like,disease%20that%20causes%20vision%20loss.

Olsen, Natalie. "Benefits of Beta Carotene and How to Get It." *Healthline*, Healthline Media, 13 Aug. 2020, https://www.healthline.com/health/beta-carotene-benefits.

Pacheco, Lorena S., et al. "Avocado Consumption and Risk of Cardiovascular Disease in US Adults." *Journal of the American Heart Association*, 30 Mar. 2022, https://www.ahajournals.org/doi/10.1161/JAHA.121.024014.

Panoff, Lauren. "The Top 10 Biotin-Rich Foods." *Healthline*, Healthline Media, 24 July 2020, https://www.healthline.com/nutrition/biotin-rich-foods.

Pearson, Keith. "Vitamin K1 vs K2: What's the Difference?" *Healthline*, Healthline Media, 15 Sept. 2017, https://www.healthline.com/nutrition/vitamin-k1-vs-k2.

Pearson, Keith. "Vitamin K1 vs K2: What's the Difference?" *Healthline*, Healthline Media, 15 Sept. 2017, https://www.healthline.com/nutrition/vitamin-k1-vs-k2.

Person. "Health Benefits of Biotin: What Does the Science Say?" *Healthline*, Healthline Media, 8 Mar. 2019, https://www.healthline.com/health/the-benefits-of-biotin.

Person. "Health Benefits of Biotin: What Does the Science Say?" *Healthline*, Healthline Media, 8 Mar. 2019, https://www.healthline.com/health/the-benefits-of-biotin.

Petre, Alina. "8 Common Signs That You're Deficient in Vitamins." *Healthline*, Healthline Media, 4 Nov. 2019, https://www.healthline.com/nutrition/vitamin-deficiency.

Petre, Alina. "Low Vitamin D and Weight Gain: Is There a Connection?" *Healthline*, Healthline Media, 7 Jan. 2021, https://www.healthline.com/nutrition/low-vitamin-d-and-weight-gain.

PF;, Jacques. "Effects of Vitamin C on High-Density Lipoprotein Cholesterol and Blood Pressure." *Journal of the American College of Nutrition*, U.S. National Library of Medicine, https://pubmed.ncbi.nlm.nih.gov/1578088/.

"Phases of the Cell Cycle (Article)." *Khan Academy*, Khan Academy, https://www.khanacademy.org/science/ap-biology/cell-communication-and-cell-cycle/cell-cycle/a/cell-cycle-phases.

"Phosphorus in Diet: Medlineplus Medical Encyclopedia." *MedlinePlus*, U.S. National Library of Medicine, https://medlineplus.gov/ency/article/002424.htm.

Pimentel, Catarina, et al. "Oxidative Stress in Alzheimer's and Parkinson's Diseases: Insights from the Yeast Saccharomyces Cerevisiae." *Oxidative Medicine and Cellular Longevity*, Hindawi Publishing Corporation, 2012, https://www.ncbi.nlm.nih.gov/pmc/articles/PMC3371773/.

Prousky, Jonathan, and Dugald Seely. "The Treatment of Migraines and Tension-Type Headaches with Intravenous and Oral Niacin (Nicotinic Acid): Systematic Review of the Literature." *Nutrition Journal*, BioMed Central, 26 Jan. 2005, https://www.ncbi.nlm.nih.gov/pmc/articles/PMC548511/.

Purdie, Jennifer. "Vitamin B-12 Deficiency and Depression: What's the Link?" *Healthline*, Healthline Media, 26 Jan. 2017, https://www.healthline.com/health/depression/b12-and-depression.

Qian, Bingjun, et al. "Effects of Vitamin B6 Deficiency on the Composition and Functional Potential of T Cell Populations." *Journal of Immunology Research*, Hindawi, 2017, https://www.ncbi.nlm.nih.gov/pmc/articles/PMC5358464/.

Rabe, Jean. "How Dogs Produce Vitamin C." *Pets on Mom.com*, 19 Nov. 2020, https://animals.mom.com/how-dogs-produce-vitamin-c-12332800.html.

Rabensteiner, Jasmin, et al. "The Impact of Folate and Vitamin B12 Status on Cognitive Function and Brain Atrophy in Healthy Elderly and Demented Austrians, a Retrospective Cohort Study." *Aging*, Impact Journals, 24 July 2020, https://www.ncbi.nlm.nih.gov/pmc/articles/PMC7467363/.

Raman, Ryan. "9 Signs and Symptoms of Copper Deficiency." *Healthline*, Healthline Media, 11 May 2018, https://www.healthline.com/nutrition/copper-deficiency-symptoms.

Raman, Ryan. "What Does Potassium Do for Your Body? A Detailed Review." *Healthline*, Healthline Media, 9 Sept. 2017, https://www.healthline.com/nutrition/what-does-potassium-do.

"Riboflavin – Vitamin B2." *The Nutrition Source*, 11 Aug. 2020, https://www.hsph.harvard.edu/nutritionsource/riboflavin-vitamin-b2/.

"Riboflavin – Vitamin B2." *The Nutrition Source*, 11 Aug. 2020, https://www.hsph.harvard.edu/nutritionsource/riboflavin-vitamin-b2/.

"Riboflavin – Vitamin B2." *The Nutrition Source*, 11 Aug. 2020, https://www.hsph.harvard.edu/nutritionsource/riboflavin-vitamin-b2/.

"Riboflavin – Vitamin B2." *The Nutrition Source*, 11 Aug. 2020, https://www.hsph.harvard.edu/nutritionsource/riboflavin-vitamin-b2/.

"Riboflavin." *Riboflavin - Health Encyclopedia - University of Rochester Medical Center*, https://www.urmc.rochester.edu/encyclopedia/content.aspx?contenttypeid=19&contentid=vitaminb-2.

Robby. "About Vitamin B5: A Guide to Usage and Dosage." *Dr. Lam Coaching - World Renowned Authority on Adrenal Fatigue Recovery*, 6 Oct. 2021, https://www.drlamcoaching.com/blog/about-vitamin-b5/.

Rogers, Kara. "Rhodopsin." *Encyclopædia Britannica*, Encyclopædia Britannica, Inc., 6 Feb. 2018, https://www.britannica.com/science/rhodopsin.

Saboor, Muhammad, et al. "Disorders Associated with Malabsorption of Iron: A Critical Review." *Pakistan Journal of Medical Sciences*, Professional Medical Publications, 2015, https://www.ncbi.nlm.nih.gov/pmc/articles/PMC4744319/.

Sarwar, Muhammad Farhan, et al. "Deficiency of Vitamin B-Complex and Its Relation with Body Disorders." *IntechOpen*, 1 Sept. 2021, https://www.intechopen.com/chapters/78374.

The Scoop on Vitamins: Vitamin B1 - Thiamine - Project Wellness. https://www.pharmaca.com/projectwellness/the-scoop-on-vitamins-vitamin-b1-thiamine/.

"Scurvy: Symptoms, Causes, Treatment, and Prevention." *Medical News Today*, MediLexicon International, https://www.medicalnewstoday.com/articles/155758.

Semeco, Arlene. "Vitamin B12 Foods: 12 Great Sources." *Healthline*, Healthline Media, 20 Jan. 2022, https://www.healthline.com/nutrition/vitamin-b12-foods.

Semeco, Arlene. "Vitamin B12 Foods: 12 Great Sources." *Healthline*, Healthline Media, 20 Jan. 2022, https://www.healthline.com/nutrition/vitamin-b12-foods.

Semeco, Arlene. "Vitamin B12 Foods: 12 Great Sources." *Healthline*, Healthline Media, 20 Jan. 2022, https://www.healthline.com/nutrition/vitamin-b12-foods.

Semeco, Arlene. "Vitamin B12 Foods: 12 Great Sources." *Healthline*, Healthline Media, 20 Jan. 2022, https://www.healthline.com/nutrition/vitamin-b12-foods.

Shaffer, Dr. Catherine. "Macrominerals and Trace Minerals in the Diet." *News*, 27 Feb. 2019, https://www.news-medical.net/health/Macrominerals-and-Trace-Minerals-in-the-Diet.aspx.

Shaffer, Dr. Catherine. "Macrominerals and Trace Minerals in the Diet." *News*, 27 Feb. 2019, https://www.news-medical.net/health/Macrominerals-and-Trace-Minerals-in-the-Diet.aspx.

Shaffer, Dr. Catherine. "Macrominerals and Trace Minerals in the Diet." *News*, 27 Feb. 2019, https://www.news-medical.net/health/Macrominerals-and-Trace-Minerals-in-the-Diet.aspx.

Sissons, Beth. "Vitamin D for Good Bone Health - Orthoinfo - Aaos." *OrthoInfo*, 22 May 2022, https://orthoinfo.aaos.org/en/staying-healthy/vitamin-d-for-good-bone-health/#:~:text=Vitamin%20D%20is%20necessary%20for,deformities%2C%20such%20as%20stooped%20posture.

"Sphingolipid." *Sphingolipid - an Overview | ScienceDirect Topics*, https://www.sciencedirect.com/topics/agricultural-and-biological-sciences/sphingolipid.

Staff, Author. "Healthy Living Guide 2021/2022." *The Nutrition Source*, 6 Jan. 2022, https://www.hsph.harvard.edu/nutritionsource/2022/01/06/healthy-living-guide-2021-2022/.

Staff, Mayo Clinic. "Iron Deficiency Anemia." *Mayo Clinic*, Mayo Foundation for Medical Education and Research, 4 Jan. 2022, https://www.mayoclinic.org/diseases-conditions/iron-deficiency-anemia/symptoms-causes/syc-20355034.

Staff, Nathan P, and Anthony J Windebank. "Peripheral Neuropathy Due to Vitamin Deficiency, Toxins, and Medications." *Continuum (Minneapolis, Minn.)*, American Academy of Neurology, Oct. 2014, https://www.ncbi.nlm.nih.gov/pmc/articles/PMC4208100/.

Streit, Lizzie. "9 Health Benefits of Vitamin B6 (Pyridoxine)." *Healthline*, Healthline Media, 1 Oct. 2018, https://www.healthline.com/nutrition/vitamin-b6-benefits#TOC_TITLE_HDR_2.

Streit, Lizzie. "9 Health Benefits of Vitamin B6 (Pyridoxine)." *Healthline*, Healthline Media, 1 Oct. 2018, https://www.healthline.com/nutrition/vitamin-b6-benefits.

Sunyecz, John A. "The Use of Calcium and Vitamin D in the Management of Osteoporosis." *Therapeutics and Clinical Risk Management*, Dove Medical Press, Aug. 2008, https://www.ncbi.nlm.nih.gov/pmc/articles/PMC2621390/.

Tarleton, Emily K., and Benjamin Littenberg. "Magnesium Intake and Depression in Adults." *American Board of Family Medicine*, American Board of Family Medicine, 1 Mar. 2015, https://www.jabfm.org/content/28/2/249.

"Thiamin – Vitamin B1." *The Nutrition Source*, 28 Oct. 2019, https://www.hsph.harvard.edu/nutritionsource/vitamin-b1/.

"Thiaminase." *Thiaminase - an Overview | ScienceDirect Topics*, https://www.sciencedirect.com/topics/biochemistry-genetics-and-molecular-biology/thiaminase.

Thompson, Liz. "Vitamin B for Skin Health & It's Benefits: Skinmindbalance." *AVEENO®*, Johnson & Johnson Consumer Inc, 1 June 2020, https://www.aveeno.com/journal/all-ways-vitamin-b-skin-sooo-good.

"Thyroid Nutrition." *Sunwarrior*, 2018-10-27 09:45:03 -0600, https://sunwarrior.com/blogs/health-hub/thyroid-nutrition.

"Tryptophan: Medlineplus Medical Encyclopedia." *MedlinePlus*, U.S. National Library of Medicine, https://medlineplus.gov/ency/article/002332.htm.

"Turnips: Health Benefits, Nutrition, and Dietary Tips." *Medical News Today*, MediLexicon International, https://www.medicalnewstoday.com/articles/284815.

UCSF Health. "Hemoglobin and Functions of Iron." *Ucsfhealth.org*, UCSF Health, 24 June 2022, https://www.ucsfhealth.org/education/hemoglobin-and-functions-of-iron.

"Vitamin A." *Mayo Clinic*, Mayo Foundation for Medical Education and Research, 13 Nov. 2020, https://www.mayoclinic.org/drugs-supplements-vitamin-a/art-20365945.

"Vitamin A: The Skincare Benefits of Retinoids: NUME-Lab." *NUME*, 23 Jan. 2022, https://www.nume-lab.com/vitamin-a-for-skin/.

"Vitamin B-12 Foods for Vegetarians and Vegans." *Medical News Today*, MediLexicon International, https://www.medicalnewstoday.com/articles/320524#foods-for-vegans.

"Vitamin B-12: Benefits, Foods, Deficiency, and Supplements." *Medical News Today*, MediLexicon International, https://www.medicalnewstoday.com/articles/219822.

"Vitamin B-12: Benefits, Foods, Deficiency, and Supplements." *Medical News Today*, MediLexicon International, https://www.medicalnewstoday.com/articles/219822.

"Vitamin B1 (Thiamine)." *Mount Sinai Health System*, https://www.mountsinai.org/health-library/supplement/vitamin-b1-thiamine.

"Vitamin B1 (Thiamine)." *Mount Sinai Health System*, https://www.mountsinai.org/health-library/supplement/vitamin-b1-thiamine.

"Vitamin B12 (Cobalamin)." *Mount Sinai Health System*, https://www.mountsinai.org/health-library/supplement/vitamin-b12-cobalamin.

"Vitamin B12 Deficiency Anemia: Medlineplus Medical Encyclopedia." *MedlinePlus*, U.S. National Library of Medicine, https://medlineplus.gov/ency/article/000574.htm.

"Vitamin B5 (Pantothenic Acid)." *Mount Sinai Health System*, https://www.mountsinai.org/health-library/supplement/vitamin-b5-pantothenic-acid.

"Vitamin B5 (Pantothenic Acid): 8 Shiitake Mushrooms (140g) A Day." *Family FECS*, 1 Jan. 1970, http://www.familyfecs.com/2016/04/vitamin-b5-pantothenic-acid-8-shiitake.html.

"Vitamin B5: Everything You Need to Know." *Medical News Today*, MediLexicon International, https://www.medicalnewstoday.com/articles/219601.

"Vitamin B5: Everything You Need to Know." *Medical News Today*, MediLexicon International, https://www.medicalnewstoday.com/articles/219601.

"Vitamin B7/Biotin: Functions, Food Sources, Deficiencies and Toxicity." *Netmeds*, https://www.netmeds.com/health-library/post/vitamin-b7-functions-food-sources-deficiencies-and-toxicity.

"Vitamin D for Good Bone Health - Orthoinfo - Aaos." *OrthoInfo*, Jan. 2020, https://orthoinfo.aaos.org/en/staying-healthy/vitamin-d-for-good-bone-health/.

"Vitamin D Metabolism and Function." *ALPCO*, 29 Nov. 2018, https://www.alpco.com/vitamin-d-metabolism-function.

"Vitamin K: Health Benefits, Daily Intake, and Sources." *Medical News Today*, MediLexicon International, https://www.medicalnewstoday.com/articles/219867.

"Vitamin." *How Products Are Made*, http://www.madehow.com/Volume-3/Vitamin.html.

"Vitamins and Minerals." *The Nutrition Source*, 25 July 2022, https://www.hsph.harvard.edu/nutritionsource/vitamins/.

"Vol 11 Issue 12 P.5-6." *American Thyroid Association*, https://www.thyroid.org/patient-thyroid-information/ct-for-patients/december-2018/vol-11-issue-12-p-5-6/.

Ware, Megan. "Copper: Health Benefits, Recommended Intake, Sources, and Risks." *Medical News Today*, MediLexicon

International, https://www.medicalnewstoday.com/articles/288165.

Ware, Megan. "Selenium: Health Benefits, Sources, and Potential Risks." *Medical News Today*, MediLexicon International, https://www.medicalnewstoday.com/articles/287842.

Ware, Meghan. "Copper: Health Benefits, Recommended Intake, Sources, and Risks." *Medical News Today*, MediLexicon International, https://www.medicalnewstoday.com/articles/288165.

Ware, Meghan. "Copper: Health Benefits, Recommended Intake, Sources, and Risks." *Medical News Today*, MediLexicon International, https://www.medicalnewstoday.com/articles/288165.

"The Water-Soluble Vitamins." *Encyclopædia Britannica*, Encyclopædia Britannica, Inc., https://www.britannica.com/science/vitamin/The-water-soluble-vitamins.

"The Water-Soluble Vitamins." *Encyclopædia Britannica*, Encyclopædia Britannica, Inc., https://www.britannica.com/science/vitamin/The-water-soluble-vitamins.

West, Helen. "6 Health Benefits of Vitamin A, Backed by Science." *Healthline*, Healthline Media, 23 Aug. 2018, https://www.healthline.com/nutrition/vitamin-a-benefits.

West, Helen. "Electrolytes: Definition, Functions, Imbalance and Sources." *Healthline*, Healthline Media, 24 Oct. 2018, https://www.healthline.com/nutrition/electrolytes.

Whelan, Corey. "Best 15 Vitamin B-6 Foods: Benefits and Recipes." *Healthline*, Healthline Media, 27 May 2017, https://www.healthline.com/health/vitamin-b6-foods.

Whelan, Corey. "Best 15 Vitamin B-6 Foods: Benefits and Recipes." *Healthline*, Healthline Media, 27 May 2017, https://www.healthline.com/health/vitamin-b6-foods.

Whelan, Corey. "What Can Vitamin A Do for Your Skin?" *Healthline*, Healthline Media, 20 Aug. 2018, https://www.healthline.com/health/beauty-skincare/vitamin-a-for-skin.

Whelan, Corey. "What Can Vitamin A Do for Your Skin?" *Healthline*, Healthline Media, 20 Aug. 2018, https://www.healthline.com/health/beauty-skincare/vitamin-a-for-skin.

Whitbread, Daisy. "Top 10 Foods Highest in Vitamin B5 (Pantothenic Acid)." *Myfooddata*, My Food Data, 23 Apr. 2022, https://www.myfooddata.com/articles/foods-high-in-pantothenic-acid-vitamin-B5.php.

Wu, Meiting, et al. "Vascular Calcification: An Update on Mechanisms and Challenges in Treatment." *Calcified Tissue International*, U.S. National Library of Medicine, Oct. 2013, https://www.ncbi.nlm.nih.gov/pmc/articles/PMC3714357/.

Yeh, Samuel D. J., and Bacon F. Chow. "Vitamin B12 Absorption in Pyridoxine-Deficient Rats: Further Studies." *OUP Academic*, Oxford University Press, 1 July 1959, https://academic.oup.com/ajcn/article-abstract/7/4/426/4730002?redirectedFrom=fulltext.

Yilma, Hagere, et al. "Is Fatigue a Cue to Obtain Iron Supplements in Odisha, India? A Mixed Methods Investigation." *BMJ Open*, BMJ Publishing Group, 20 Oct. 2020, https://www.ncbi.nlm.nih.gov/pmc/articles/PMC7577027/.

"Your Teeth Are Made of These Three Layers Dental Anatomy 101." *Teeth Are Made of THESE Three Layers | Asleep For Dentistry*, http://www.asleepfordentistry.com/blog/three-layers-of-a-tooth.html.

Zelman, Contributors: Kathleen. "Iodine a Critically Important Nutrient." *EatRight*, 1 Apr. 2021, https://www.eatright.org/food/vitamins-and-supplements/types-of-vitamins-and-nutrients/iodine-a-critically-important-nutrient.

Zheng, Wei, and Andrew D Monnot. "Regulation of Brain Iron and Copper Homeostasis by Brain Barrier Systems: Implication in Neurodegenerative Diseases." *Pharmacology & Therapeutics*, U.S. National Library of Medicine, Feb. 2012, https://www.ncbi.nlm.nih.gov/pmc/articles/PMC3268876/.

Made in the USA
Las Vegas, NV
23 March 2025